Patrick Holford BSc, DipION, FBANT is a leading spokesman on nutrition in the media, specialising in the field of mental health. He is the author of over 40 books, translated into over 30 languages and selling millions of copies worldwide, including *The Optimum Nutrition Bible*, *The Low GL Diet Bible*, *The Hybrid Diet* and *Flu Fighters*.

Patrick Holford started his academic career in the field of psychology. In 1984 he founded the Institute for Optimum Nutrition (ION), an independent educational charity, with his mentor, twice Nobel Prize winner Dr Linus Pauling, as patron. ION has been researching and helping to define what it means to be optimally nourished for the past 25 years and is one of the most respected educational establishments for training nutritional therapists. At ION Patrick was involved in ground-breaking research showing that multivitamins can increase children's IQ scores – the subject of a *Horizon* documentary in the 1980s. He was one of the first promoters of the importance of zinc, antioxidants, essential fats, low-GL diets and homocysteine-lowering B vitamins, as well as vitamin C for fighting flu.

He is also founder of the Food for the Brain Foundation. He is in the Orthomolecular Medicine Hall of Fame and is an honorary fellow of the British Association for Nutrition and Lifestyle Medicine, as well a Complementary and Natural Healthcare registered practitioner.

patrick
HOLFORD

OPTIMUM
NUTRITION
FOR
VEGANS

How to be healthy and optimally nourished on a plant-based diet

PIATKUS

PIATKUS

First published in Great Britain in 2020 by Piatkus

1 3 5 7 9 10 8 6 4 2

A CIP catalogue record for this book
is available from the British Library.

ISBN 978-0-349-42581-8

Typeset in Minion by M Rules
Printed and bound in Great Britain by
Clays Ltd, Elcograf S.p.A

Papers used by Piatkus are from well-managed forests
and other responsible sources.

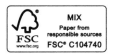

MIX
Paper from
responsible sources
FSC® C104740
FSC www.fsc.org

Piatkus
An imprint of
Little, Brown Book Group
Carmelite House
50 Victoria Embankment
London EC4Y 0DZ

An Hachette UK Company
www.hachette.co.uk

www.littlebrown.co.uk

Note: some of the recipes in this book have previously appeared in
The 10 Secrets of 100% Health Cookbook, *Food GLorious Food*,
The Low-GL Diet Cookbook or *The Perfect Pregnancy Cookbook*.

Acknowledgements

My role in writing this book was to sift through the latest research on topics relevant to a vegan diet and turn it into practical advice for all. To that end I am grateful to Martyn Hooper of the Pernicious Anaemia Society for his tireless work digging deep into vitamin B12; to the Vegan Society, and especially Heather Russell, for providing scientific resources for so many vegan issues; to Captain Joseph Hibbeln and Professor Michael Crawford for their excellent work on omega-3 fats and their role in human health; to Dr William Grant for his help with the science relating to vitamin D; to Jazz and Lola Mellor for their practical advice on all things vegan; to Fiona McDonald Joyce for her fantastic recipes; and to my wife Gaby, who explored and helped me try out many of the delicious recipes and principles in this book.

Disclaimer

Although all the nutrients and dietary changes referred to in this book have been proven safe, those seeking help for specific medical conditions are advised to consult a qualified nutrition therapist, clinical nutritionist, doctor or equivalent health professional. The recommendations given in this book are solely intended as education and information, and should not be taken as medical advice. Neither the author nor the publisher accept liability for readers who choose to self-prescribe.

Contents

Part 3

Introduction

How to be a Healthy Vegan

There are many compelling reasons for becoming vegan, ranging from ethical concerns about animals and the need to reduce meat consumption for low-carbon living, to personal choice: perhaps it's the food you like and you feel good eating it. Whatever your reasons, my purpose in this book is to make sure that you do it in a way that will optimise your health and that of your family. I want you to be a super-healthy vegan.

In 1984 I founded the Institute for Optimum Nutrition with the purpose of researching what kind of food and diet might be the key to optimal health, and to train nutritional therapists. In those early days I set our nutrition students an assignment, which was to become vegan for a week – so no meat, fish, eggs or dairy products. I did this myself for over a year. Many people experienced substantial improvements in their health and learnt how to expand their repertoire of foods, menus and meals to accommodate the reduction they now had in their food choices. There were very few packaged or pre-prepared foods that would tick the vegan box in those days and next to nothing that one could eat in restaurants, so we discovered how to make a rich and tasty variety of dishes from vegan ingredients.

This resulted in a library of delicious vegan recipes (shared with you in Part 3) that also achieved our goal of optimum nutrition. These recipes embrace the optimum nutrition principles that I outline in Part 1, which, when combined with the practical guidance in this book, explains how you can achieve optimum vegan nutrition. So you will discover both *why* it's important to eat certain foods and food combinations and *how* to make them a part of your diet.

For those new to the concept of 'optimum nutrition', it is based on first establishing what optimal health *is*. I defined this in 1998, in my book *The Optimum Nutrition Bible*, as not only freedom from disease but also as having an abundance of energy, mental clarity and good mood, and an absence of niggling problems – for example, those that affect digestion, hormone balance or the skin – and an ability to perform physically at peak, as has been demonstrated by numerous vegan athletes. In that bestselling book, I considered all the evidence for the type of diet and nutrient intake that would allow us to function at our peak, both for physical health and psychological health and happiness. I also considered what our ancestors would have eaten, especially during critical phases in our evolution linked, for example, to increases in brain size.

About 6 million years ago our hominid ancestors split from other primate apes such as chimpanzees and gorillas. Despite having essentially the same genome – we share 98.5 per cent of the same genes – the brain size of those early humans gradually increased until about 100,000 years ago when *Homo sapiens* emerged with a brain size three times that of other primates. Our brain is what makes us human, therefore there's a good argument that we should set our optimal intake of nutrients to whatever is optimal for brain function.

These fundamental principles of optimum nutrition are explained in Chapter 1, which provides the *raison d'être* for following a more plant-based diet (Chapter 2). You'll also see how nutrients are team players (Chapter 3) and why the baseline for health is whole, organic and unadulterated food. In fact, many of today's endemic diseases are not just a consequence of sub-optimum nutrition but also the result of the deluge of anti-nutrients (substances we take in from food, drink or air that have a negative effect on our health). We cannot avoid being exposed to many of these; however, there are diet and lifestyle changes that minimise your exposure to harmful chemicals and pollution in your food, water and air. This is explored and explained in Chapter 4, Anti-Nutrients – the Dark Side of Nutrition.

You will learn that it is not possible to get all the nutrients you need for optimal health from a strictly vegan diet, hence the need to supplement some of them. In addition, there are some nutrients that it is difficult to achieve in sufficient levels from *any* diet – vitamin D in the winter months being a good example. We will explore the nutrients that are either impossible or very hard to obtain through a vegan diet, and your options for achieving an optimum intake. These include vitamins B12 and D (Chapter 8), and omega-3 fats and phospholipids, notably DHA and choline (Chapter 6). Exactly what it is advisable to supplement is explained in Chapter 11.

You can get enough of the macro-nutrients (protein, carbohydrates and fats) providing that you eat the right foods in the correct amounts and combinations, which is particularly relevant to protein (which is discussed in Chapter 5). With carbohydrates, the danger is in eating too many fast-releasing carbs (and sugar), which are often found in pre-prepared vegan foods and snacks, so how to control your carbs and your energy is the subject of Chapter 7. I will also explore the role of fat, and the essential fats such as omega-3, omega-6 and phospholipids, in Chapter 6.

Although I won't go into too much detail on the ethical and

ecological arguments for plant-based diets, these are addressed in the part of the book that covers how to achieve optimum nutrition. These arguments are important because, in most cases, protecting your own health is very much connected to protecting animals and the planet. The ideal position is one of no compromise – in other words to find a way to eat that is optimal for you and your family, all animals and the eco-system. But there are, inevitably, some tension points and elements of personal choice. Where these exist I will highlight them, not in order to tell you what to do but to let you know about the relevant issues from a nutritional point of view so that you can make an informed choice.

If you follow the advice, and the recipes, in this book you will be able to eat an exclusively plant-based diet without compromising your health at all. Indeed, as a consequence, you will experience increased vitality and greater freedom from the diseases associated with the classic Western diet that is high in meat, dairy and processed foods. You will also be eating a carbon-friendly, humane diet.

Wishing you the best of health,

Patrick Holford

Part 1

The Foundations of Optimum Nutrition

What is optimum nutrition? Quite simply, it is whatever nutrition is needed for optimal health – essentially, to feel great and to be free from disease. You'll learn that a largely plant-based diet is essential to achieve this and that there is a complex web of nutrients in whole foods that also help to protect us from the ever-increasing deluge of anti-nutrients: pollutants in food, water and air that are changing what we need in the way of nutrition in order to stay healthy.

Chapter 1

The Principles of Optimum Nutrition

B efore diving into how to be a healthy vegan, it's important to define what 'healthy' means and the fundamental principles of optimum nutrition, which I'll be applying to a vegan diet.

There's an outdated view that the aim of nutrition is to ensure that we get enough vitamins, minerals, protein and fats in order to function without any obvious deficiency diseases, such as rickets (vitamin D deficiency) or scurvy (vitamin C deficiency). That's the basis of the original recommended daily allowances (RDAs – or, as I call them, ridiculous dietary arbitraries), which are now called reference nutrient intakes (RNIs). They serve a purpose, but they represent a very low yardstick. They do not aim for *optimum* nutrition.

I want you to be super-healthy, full of energy, with lots of disease resilience so that you can shake off a cold quickly and rise to the challenge of life's inevitable stresses. For that you need *optimum* nutrition.

When I started researching this topic back in the 1980s at the Institute for Optimum Nutrition (ION), the first thing we needed was a yardstick of optimal health. Our working definition was:

- Optimum physical function
- Optimum psychological function
- Optimum chemical function
- Absence of ill-health – signs and symptoms
- Longevity – longest healthy lifespan

We looked at studies on athletes, marathon runners, IQ, mood, memory and so on. We wanted to find out what were the optimal intakes of nutrients that would get a marathon runner running faster or would increase IQ: for example, I worked with one professional cyclist, Mick Ballard, who was ranked the tenth fastest, but within months of optimising his nutrient intake he went to number one and stayed in the lead for several years, which he attributed to optimum nutrition.

At the Institute for Optimum Nutrition we studied a group of 90 schoolchildren, aged 12 to 13, giving them an optimum multivitamin and mineral versus a placebo. Only those on the multi had a significant seven-point increase in IQ score. This study was filmed by the *Horizon* team on BBC television and published in the *Lancet* medical journal.[1]) It was the first randomised, placebo-controlled trial showing how an increased intake of nutrients can improve intelligence, highlighting the need to consider the brain when setting optimum nutrient levels.

The research led to the creation of a questionnaire, the 100% Health Check, which shows you how healthy you are out of 100 per cent (see Resources). If you woke up tomorrow 100 per cent healthy how would you know? Think about it. You could probably write down two or three measurable things – perhaps your energy would be increased, you'd experience emotional balance when stressed, improved digestion, lack of aches and pains, that kind of thing. Now score yourself out of ten, where ten is the best and zero is the worst. What score do you give yourself for energy? Let's say, for example, it was 5. Write this down and date it. As you improve your nutrition, with diet and supplements, check in with yourself and re-score your energy, then see what happens. In this way you can work out optimum nutrition for yourself through your own personal experimentation.

In our research we defined optimum nutrition as the level that:

- Promotes optimal physical function.
- Promotes optimal psychological function.
- Promotes optimal chemical function.
- Is associated with the lowest incidence of disease.
- Is associated with the longest healthy lifespan.
- Is consistent with evolutionary and animal models.

The first two are easy to understand with my earlier examples of an athlete's performance and children's IQ. Chemical function means having good scores for the indicators of health, such as your blood homocysteine level (which you'll understand when we talk about B vitamins, especially B12) and markers of inflammation or cholesterol. These are chemical measures that show what's going on in your body.

One thing that I became aware of is that for every disease that exists there's a country that doesn't have it. Southern Asian countries, including China and Thailand, have an exceptionally low incidence of breast and prostate cancer, with 25 times less prostate cancer incidence and a fraction of the mortality[2] and five times less breast cancer[3] than Western nations.

The Japanese have the lowest rate of dementia.[4] Many African countries with more traditional diets have a fraction of the diabetes incidence compared to the UK's 7 per cent (or 4.7 million diabetics)[5], or the USA's 11 per cent of the population[6]. By studying what's different in the diet of countries with the lowest risk of certain diseases, I've been able to tease out the key attributes for optimum nutrition.

As you'll see in the next chapter, many diseases are less common in people and countries that have a more plant-based or vegetarian diet. There are not so many surveys that separate vegan from vegetarian diets, however, and there are quite a few studies that show that pescatarians (people who avoid meat but eat fish) also do very well. What vegans, vegetarians and pescatarians tend to have in common, however, is a highly plant-based diet.

Building your health resilience

Diseases don't come out of nowhere. They happen when you lose your health resilience, which you could think of as the balance in your 'health deposit account'. Too often, when someone is diagnosed with diabetes after a period of stress, or they develop breast or prostate cancer after eating a diet high in dairy for many years, or when an elderly parent develops dementia after their partner dies, the disease is blamed on that one factor. But it's usually just the final straw that broke the camel's back. Of course, stress, loss and diet all impact your health, but if you have enough health resilience you can roll with the punches of life without succumbing to disease. In contrast, when you're 'overdrawn' in your health deposit account, disease is just around the corner.

Let's explore how this works to understand what optimum nutrition truly means and why it helps to define what to eat for health more clearly than the conventional approach of 'getting enough' nutrients to prevent obvious deficiencies. Even the word 'deficiency', which means lack of efficiency, shows why the optimum nutrition approach is the right way to think. I am interested, both for my own sake and for yours, in how to help our bodies and minds to be efficient. If people who take in a certain amount of vitamin C have fewer or shorter colds, then it would seem that their immune systems are obviously more efficient. They have more *resilience* – more money in that health deposit account. You don't want to feel only 'all right'; you want to feel vibrant, full of energy and disease-proof. That's what optimum nutrition is all about.

The new model of health

Instead of thinking of the body as a machine, and disease as a spanner in the works that must be destroyed or removed with drugs or surgery, medical scientists are now beginning to look at human beings as a complex adaptive system, more like a self-organising jungle or eco-system. This necessitates understanding the big picture, including our interaction with diet and the environment as drivers of disease, as opposed to focusing on one element and treating the body like a complicated computer (for example, blocking an enzyme or manipulating a gene), in a similar way to a software programmer adjusting a bit of code.

Rather than trying to control a person's health by playing God with hi-tech medicine and genetic manipulation, the optimum-nutrition approach of looking at health considers a human being as a whole, with an interconnected mind and body designed to adapt to health if the circumstances are right. A classic example of this has been the approach to the coronavirus. While mainstream medicine has focused on finding a drug or a vaccine, an optimum nutrition approach would also consider how our innately intelligent immune system can be supported to fight off the virus. Vaccines are much more effective in those with the most resilient immune systems, so these approaches are not mutually exclusive. That's why older people, with less efficient immune systems, have the least benefit from yearly flu vaccines, which are rated to be between 10 (2017–18) and 34 (2018–19) per cent effective in the 65-plus age group.[7] In addition, the problem with most vaccines, and drugs, is that they introduce anti-nutrients into the body that are difficult for the body to detoxify.

The new model of health

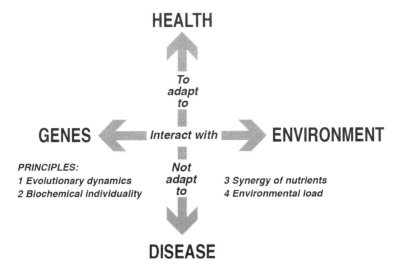

Your genes interact with your environment (that is, everything you eat, drink and breathe) to create you. If you have good nutrition, the result is that you have the capacity to adapt to the stresses of life – that's health. If your total environmental load exceeds your genetic capacity to adapt, you develop disease.

Of course, this adaptive capacity is not the same for everyone. We are each born with different strengths and weaknesses, and varying levels of resilience. Some of us have what is popularly called 'good genes' or we come from 'good stock', and some of us do not. According to this new concept, our health is a result of the interaction between our inherited adaptive capacity and our circumstances. On a physical/chemical level, for example, that interaction would be between our genes and our environment. If our environment is sufficiently hostile (through bad diet, pollution, exposure to viruses, allergens and so on) we exceed our ability to adapt and we get sick.

Nature or nurture? The interplay of genes and environment

One of the ongoing debates in the study of health today is whether our genes (nature) or our environment (nurture) define who we are and how healthy we will be. Of course, it's both. Furthermore, your environment, of which your diet is the most direct part, changes the activity of your genes. This is the new science of epigenetics ('epi' means 'upon' – the effects of your environment on your genetic expression). Environment is the bigger influence on health. This is illustrated by studies of genetically identical twins. Do they get the same diseases? In these studies, hereditability accounts for roughly 20 per cent of disease risk, thus 80 per cent can be attributed to environment.[8] But hereditability doesn't refer only to genes, because these identical twins share lots of common factors in their environments and upbringing. The genes you inherit are much less predictive of the diseases you'll suffer with than what you put in your mouth. We are, on the whole, digging our own graves with a knife and fork.

Cancer is a case in point. One in three people in the Western world have a cancer diagnosis during their lifetime. When I was born in 1958 it was less than one in ten. That's a clear indication that whatever we've done to our overall environment in the developed world, whether it is what we eat, breathe or drink, or the chemicals or radiation we expose ourselves to (which includes mobile phones and ever-increasing exposure to electromagnetic radiation from Wi-Fi signals), plus our state of mind and levels of stress, has exceeded our cells' capacity to stay healthy. While it can be argued that improved cancer screening is bound to uncover more cases, and thus increase the incidence, better treatment should lead to lower mortality, yet the five-year survival rate from breast cancer, once diagnosed, has only increased from 49 per cent in 1970 to 54 per cent, while incidence of the disease has increased by over 50 per cent.[9] As we introduce these potential stressors it is absolutely right that we need, first, to test their effects on our health.

We already know that the risk of cancer is increased if we smoke, regularly drink excess alcohol, eat red and processed meat and dairy produce, take certain drugs and hormones, are exposed to exhaust fumes and other pollutants, or have used mobile phones for ten years or more – to name a few. On the other hand, the risk is lower if we have a high intake of certain vegetables, fibres, antioxidant vitamins, such as vitamin C, and live in an unpolluted environment. Evidence shows that, when the pluses significantly outweigh the minuses, health can be improved. That's also why vegans, who (a) eat more veg, antioxidants and fibre, and (b) avoid meat and milk, have a much lower cancer risk (as I will explain in the next chapter).

Antioxidants and free radicals

Our life depends on oxygen. We generate energy 'combusting' glucose with oxygen and, in the process, create the equivalent of exhaust fumes called free oxidising radicals, often abbreviated to free radicals or oxidants. These damage our cells in much the same way that oxidants in the air rust metal or make a cut apple go brown. That 'oxidation' process is disarmed by antioxidants, which are nutrients such as vitamins A, C and E that can neutralise these harmful oxidants.

How our environment affects our genes

Our genes and the environment are like the chicken and the egg: science is proving that our genes are influenced by the environment in which we have evolved and that the environment also affects our genes throughout our life. More recently, science is showing how the environment we expose our genes to, be it diet or chemical exposure for example, instructs our genes to behave in a certain way. For example, we might be genetically inclined towards heart problems but it is our environment (what we eat, whether we smoke, the exercise we take and where we live) that determines whether those heart problems will develop. Through studying this, we have learnt that our genetic programming is not set in stone, but that genes, which are the instructions to make things like enzymes or hormones, are more like dimmer switches that can be turned up or down. This is called 'gene expression' and it is the key to the new area of science called epigenetics that I mentioned earlier: outside influences turn gene messages up or down.

An example is the BRCA gene, which, if you have it, increases your risk of breast cancer. Roughly half those with the BRCA gene develop breast cancer during their lifetime. But half don't. Why the difference? One possible reason is that a high intake of dairy products raises a growth hormone called IGF-1, which makes breast cancer cells grow. According to Professor Jeff Holly, from Bristol University's Faculty of Medicine, one of the world's leading experts in IGF, 'Those in the top quarter for blood IGF-1 levels have approximately a three to fourfold increase in risk of breast, prostate or colorectal cancer.' On the other hand, soya dampens down the BRCA gene, making developing breast cancer less likely.[10]

Similarly, how we interact with our environment – for example, our ability to digest certain nutrients – depends on our genetic make-up. Some people simply don't make enough of the enzymes that digest beans or greens, for example, therefore these foods cause them to bloat and become gaseous. If they were to supplement the enzymes that digest these foods – called amyloglucosidase and alpha-galactosidase, respectively – the problem would be solved.

In my opinion, the future of medicine might focus primarily on genetics and on environmental medicine, of which nutrition plays a major part, as the means to influence health – this is sometimes called functional medicine. Genes are harder to change than diet, so the role of nutrition becomes even more important in this kind of approach to healthcare, along with strategies to reduce anti-nutrients, which include substances such as environmental pollutants, pesticides and chemical food additives – these all interfere with the beneficial action of nutrients (see Chapter 4). I hope that the vegan movement will not solely be about not eating animal products but, much like the approach taken by the organic movement, will also include the principles of avoiding, or at least limiting, these anti-nutrients in food.

Remember that our health is always being challenged – be it as the result of a partner's or colleague's cold or unavoidable exhaust fumes. What we take into our bodies – whether healthy food, drink, drugs or junk food – can dramatically affect our ability to stay healthy. It's a balancing act in which we aim to eat, drink and breathe what is necessary to add to our *adaptive* capacity, and to minimise those elements that rob us of *resilience*. As well as thinking of these negative elements as anti-nutrients, we can also view them as anti-adaptogens (negative environmental factors that work against our adaptive capacity).

A new way of thinking – the development of modern medicine

The birth of modern science and medicine is often said to emanate from the Age of Reason in the 17th and 18th centuries. Partly as a reaction to superstitious medieval Europe, we entered the era of Newton and other scientists who could eloquently show cause and effect in natural phenomena by means of experiments. As important as this scientific revolution has been, it had, and still has, a downside. Many vital parts of life, such as emotions and spirituality, couldn't be measured in a scientific way and became increasingly less important in Western culture.

The belief was (and still is to a large extent) that by running precise experiments on, for example, small pieces of our biology, we would discover the secret of health. This approach is called 'reductionism', in that you reduce a complex system into tiny pieces, which you then examine in detail, in the belief that you'll understand the whole by putting all the pieces of the jigsaw together. Intellect triumphed – science became dominant over art and God, and today there is a cultural belief that science will solve humankind's ills. Science is the new religion. 'We are led by the science' say our governments, while ignoring the science of nutrition.

The apparent failure of modern medicine to stem the tide of cancer (now affecting one in three people at some point in their life, as we saw earlier), diabetes (present in one in six people over the age of 40), and other debilitating and largely preventable diseases such as dementia – where only 1 per cent of the risk is attributed to genes[11] – bears testimony to the fact that the reductionist approach is not good for understanding complex living systems, such as ourselves. Either that or medicine has been largely hijacked by the pharmaceutical industry and nutrition has been purposely sidelined. In reality, it's a bit of both.

Reductionist thinking is still the dominant approach in modern medicine, culminating in the randomised placebo-controlled trial (RCT), where one group is given a dummy pill and the other the drug being tested. This approach, which looks at a drug as the answer for all disease, although great for the drug industry, is ultimately bad for your health because it has skewed modern medicine towards drugs and away from diet and lifestyle factors, which don't lend themselves so easily to RCTs. How do you conduct, for example, an RCT on a vegan diet?

The research bar has purposely been raised so high, and the hoops you have to jump through are so difficult and heavily influenced by the pharma/medical community, that the cost of the average 'high-quality' RCT is seven million dollars, making it a game that generally only drug companies and governments can play. But governments, for the large part, don't fund nutrition studies so in the end there's a lack of research.

Building your health resilience

The reductionist/RCT way of doing science is not the only, or the best, way to do science, and, as you'll see, a new systems-based science is emerging that truly gives us insight into how to reverse today's health issues and achieve a high level of good health. It starts by looking at the whole system, the big picture – in this case, us human beings – and the fundamental factors that determine our state of health. A fundamental part of systems thinking is the concept of 'resilience' that I mentioned earlier.

A taxi driver called John once said to me, 'I used to be fine, then suddenly I have diabetes. What's that about?' In systems thinking one would depict John's previous state of apparently stable health, which no doubt fluctuated somewhat from day to day, by the position of a ball in the 'basin of health', shown in the diagram below. His state of health is held in place by a number of criteria, such as his intake of sugar and refined carbohydrates, his stress level, his degree of insulin resistance (a result of losing control of blood sugar), a lack of exercise and his alcohol consumption. When enough of these conditions had eventually reduced our taxi driver's resilience to zero, his health tipped into a new, relatively stable, but unhealthy, state: the basin called diabetes.

The resilience model of health

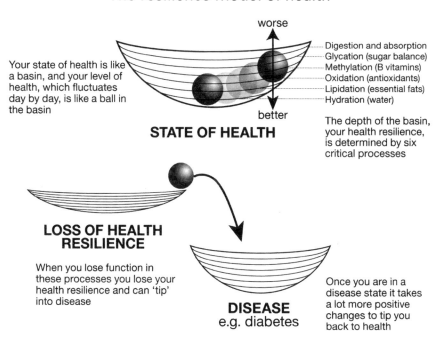

worse

Your state of health is like a basin, and your level of health, which fluctuates day by day, is like a ball in the basin

Digestion and absorption
Glycation (sugar balance)
Methylation (B vitamins)
Oxidation (antioxidants)
Lipidation (essential fats)
Hydration (water)

better

STATE OF HEALTH

The depth of the basin, your health resilience, is determined by six critical processes

LOSS OF HEALTH RESILIENCE

When you lose function in these processes you lose your health resilience and can 'tip' into disease

DISEASE
e.g. diabetes

Once you are in a disease state it takes a lot more positive changes to tip you back to health

Another finding in systems-based science is that you need much more extreme changes to tip yourself *back* into good health: for example, we all need about 50mcg (micrograms) of the essential mineral chromium a day to help keep blood sugar levels stable, because this nutrient makes the hormone insulin work properly. You could eat almost that quantity with a wholefood diet.

If you've developed diabetes, however, like our taxi driver John, you need *500mcg* a day – ten times the usual amount – to help to reverse it. Simply eating a well-balanced diet might help to prevent diabetes, but it won't *reverse* it (and yes, you *can* reverse type-2 diabetes, the common kind). To reverse diabetes you have to follow a strict no-sugar, low-carb diet and, ideally, supplement with high-dose chromium, more than you would ever achieve from your diet, until your blood sugar level becomes stable and you are declared diabetes-free.

The same is true with vitamin C: you need much more when you're under viral attack. Taking 6g (grams), or more, of vitamin C in the first day of a cold is consistently shown to shorten the duration and severity; for example, in a study giving 8g a day, 46 per cent of participants were symptom-free within 24 hours.[12] When you're sick, you need more nutrients to get well. If you were to try to obtain 6g of vitamin C from oranges you would have to eat over 100, so you cannot achieve these levels with diet alone.

The six secrets of optimum nutrition

One common finding arising out of systems-based studies of complex adaptive systems, whether applied to economies, ecologies or our bodies, is that there are usually only half a dozen critical factors that keep the system healthy. Eating a more plant-based diet is one such factor that is vital to keep our 'ecological systems' healthy.

The vast majority of the diseases and health problems we suffer with are a consequence of losing our resilience or adaptability in one or more of only six fundamental core biological processes. Bringing these six processes back into balance is the best way to build your health resilience.

As I will explain later, it is what you *digest and absorb*, not just what you *eat*, that determines your health. Every cell and every chemical reaction inside your body depends, second by second, on what you eat and how you digest and absorb it. The first secret of optimum nutrition is to optimise your ability to digest and absorb the nutrients you consume, and to eat the correct diet, and to take the right supplements.

The next five fundamental processes are called glycation, methylation, oxidation, lipidation and hydration. In layman's terms, these relate to:

- How we process carbohydrates, which is the subject of Chapter 7.
- How B vitamins turn your food into energy and act as catalysts through a process called methylation (there are a billion methylation reactions in your brain and body every few seconds) – this is covered in Chapter 8.
- How essential fats help our cells communicate with each other and keep us physically, mentally and emotionally healthy – this is covered in Chapter 6.
- How we make our own exhaust fumes (waste), called oxidants, and how we disarm those oxidants with antioxidants – this is covered in Chapter 2.
- And the vital role of water, the body's most abundant nutrient. While vital, the message here is very simple: drink eight glasses of good-quality water a day. That means filtered water. Mineral water is good, but we don't want more plastic bottles in our environment.

How to reverse internal global warming

You could think of losing function in the critical processes described above as your own internal global warming. Of course, you can't reverse this by just taking a drug. That's as ridiculous as trying to save the polar bear by giving it a drug to lower its body temperature. You have to change the whole ecosystem, in the case of your body by changing what you put into your mouth. Eating a plant-based diet is a great way to start but, even so, there are some nutrients such as vitamin B12, the omega-3 fat DHA and phospholipids that it isn't really possible to get enough of on a purely vegan diet. I'll let you know what to do about those in Chapters 6 and 8.

Fortunately, it's much easier to reverse internal global warming in your body than the global warming of the planet. Given that more than half your entire body is replaced each year by the natural renewal of cells, and this is achieved from the nutrients in your food, you can turn your body's ecology round in months, not years.

Why supplements are essential

One of the biggest myths in nutrition is that you can get all the vitamins you need from a well-balanced diet. If you ask, 'What is a well-balanced diet?' however, the retort is usually 'A diet that gives you all the vitamins you need.' If you ask what 'need' means, you're given the RDA or RNI levels (see page 7), which are simply the lowest levels required (with a bit of a safety margin built in) to stop the effects of chronic deficiency, such as the bowed legs of vitamin D deficiency (rickets) or the crashing immune system, bleeding and gum degeneration of vitamin C deficiency (scurvy).

Let's take vitamins C and D as an example. You need only 40mg (milligrams) of vitamin C a day to prevent scurvy. The RNI is 80mg a day, so you could double this just to be on the safe side; however, levels of 500mg a day *dramatically* reduce the risk of heart disease, and an intake of 1,000mg a day reduces the risk of cancer. And, as we have seen, 6,000mg (6g), or more, during the first day of an infection such as a cold or flu optimises your chances of a faster recovery with less severe symptoms.

The RNI of vitamin D was 5mcg in the past, which is enough

to prevent rickets. Like vitamin C, the RNI has been doubled to 10mcg (400iu – international units) as a 'just-in-case' measure. Is this optimal? No. People who have higher intakes, or with higher blood levels of vitamin D, suffer with less heart disease, cancer and viral infections. You probably need to supplement 25mcg (1,000iu) vitamin D to be close to optimum, as well as getting regular sun exposure. I supplement 15mcg (600iu) in the summer and 25mcg (1,000iu) in the winter.

You could, of course, argue that vitamin C is special because we primates have lost the ability to make it, so we need to eat or supplement more, and that vitamin D supplementation is a consequence of living far from the equator (humanity's original habitat), living indoors and wearing clothes. But there's a much simpler explanation as to why we need to supplement: we don't eat enough. This is certainly true for most essential vitamins, minerals and essential fats.

Our changing diet

Before there were cars and fridges our ancestors had to walk to gather and hunt food, fetch water and chop wood. All food was organic and whole. Good food goes off, so you have to eat it fresh, all of which means more nutrients. Even in the mid-Victorian era the average man was expending 3,000–4,500 calories per day and women were expending 2,400–3,500 calories per day.[13] Today the average man consumes 2,500 calories and the average woman 2,000 calories – and they are gaining weight. Therefore, our ancestors not only had more nutrient-rich food, they also ate almost twice as much quantity. A report by the Royal Society of Medicine concludes: 'since it would be unacceptable and impracticable to recreate the high calorie mid-Victorian working class diet, this constitutes either a persuasive argument for a more widespread use of food fortification and/or food supplements'.

Ninety-nine point nine per cent of humanity's history, and

most of its evolution up to 10,000 years ago when brain size reached its zenith, has occurred eating a diet rich in plants, fish and, occasionally, meat. It is therefore reasonable to assume that we evolved to use and need the nutrients that would have been available to us then, not just what the average diet of the past 100 years provides. Fruit and veg intake is an example. While five servings of fruit and veg is the mantra of governments, seven equates to a lower risk of disease and, according to a study pooling the results of 95 surveys by Imperial College London, eating ten servings a day could prevent 7.8 million premature deaths each year .[14] But modern humans, unlike a primate in the wild, would get fat eating ten servings of carb-rich fruit and veg. Twice Nobel Prize winner Dr Linus Pauling worked out that we need 2g of vitamin C a day, roughly half that of a gorilla, which is twice our weight at 150kg. If you want to be in optimal good health, not average poor health, you need to take supplements as well as eating a wholefood diet, rich in plant foods.

Your quick guide to the principles of optimum nutrition

The principles of optimum nutrition provide a new yardstick for defining an *optimal* diet, not one solely based on preventing obvious deficiency diseases.

- Optimum nutrition is defined as whatever intake of a nutrient, or type of diet, promotes optimal health as well as a lower incidence of disease.
- Since we are exposed to many anti-nutrients – factors in our diet, environment and lifestyle that increase our need for nutrients – these must be minimised.

- Optimum nutrition has a direct and positive effect on genetic expression. What you eat has a much larger influence on your health than the genes you are born with.
- Disease results from a loss of resilience, or adaptive capacity, which can be restored by increasing your intake of nutrients and reducing your intake of anti-nutrients.

Chapter 2

Choosing a More Plant-Based Diet Makes Good Health Sense

You can be a healthy or an unhealthy vegan, just the same as meat-eaters can be healthy or unhealthy. The longest living tribe we know of is the Tsimané tribe in the Peruvian Amazon, who have the lowest risk of heart disease in the world. They eat a high-carb diet comprising 72 per cent of calories from unrefined, high-fibre carbohydrates, such as rice, plantain, manioc, corn, nuts and fruits. Protein makes up 14 per cent of their diet, mainly from lean animal meat and fish, largely wild pigs, piranha and catfish. Don't worry, I'm not going to suggest that you follow their example, but I am going to show you how to get this much protein directly from vegan sources in Chapter 5.

The fat intake of the Tsimané tribe is low at 14 per cent, which is much less than a Western diet, and even those over the age of 75 have virtually no heart disease or hardening of the arteries. They also burn off a lot of calories from exercise, so they need to eat more carbohydrate. The average man spends six or seven hours, and the average woman four to five hours, being physically active: hunting, gathering and preparing land for farming. If you do no exercise, this amount of carbohydrate, as I will show you in Chapter 7, will make you fat.

Apart from the health benefits, there are many important and legitimate environmental, ecological and humanitarian reasons to go largely or wholly vegan. This is not my area of focus in this book, nor my area of speciality, but there are two overarching principles that tie in with health food and farming that make total sense.

The world's climate and your own personal environment

Life can be reflected by two overlapping cycles. These are the cycles of oxygen and carbon. We, and all animals, are oxygen-based life forms. We 'burn' carbon-based carbohydrates with the oxygen we breathe in and generate 'exhaust fumes' called oxidants. Technically these oxidants are called ROSs (reactive oxygen species), meaning that they are dangerous, unstable forms of spent oxygen. Once the oxygen we breathe in has done its energy-generating work, we breathe out carbon dioxide. When we burn carbon-based fossil fuels they release larger quantities of carbon dioxide and, in some cases, carbon monoxide. These absorb heat and create a 'greenhouse' effect, contributing to global warming. The carbon that is captured in the soil and plants as they grow is released into the atmosphere when we burn wood and fossil fuels, and eat carbohydrate. The same is true of animals eating vegetation. All this accelerates global warming. Plants and trees are key because they absorb carbon dioxide and monoxide, using it to grow, and when they decay, return that carbon back into the soil.

To counteract global warming you have to capture carbon, and turn oxides into oxygen, which is what trees and plants do.

To reiterate, they take in carbon monoxide and carbon dioxide, capture the carbon, and make oxygen, which is essential for all life forms. The carbon is incorporated into the plant's structure as carbohydrate (carbon, hydrogen and oxygen trapped together by the sun's energy), which we then 'burn' when we eat the carbohydrate, thereby releasing the sun's trapped energy – and then the cycle goes around again.

The biggest sources of carbon capture are soil and trees. Tiny organisms in the soil help to capture carbon, making topsoil. The destruction of soil by deep ploughing in industrialised agriculture, releases carbon. Therefore, every time another 1,000 acres of rainforest is chopped down to graze cattle, or to grow soya to feed animals or humans, that represents less carbon capture. Having mixed farming, where there is grazing and thus production of manure, is also essential to maintaining topsoil.

Micro-organisms such as the magnificent *Emiliania huxleyi* (a form of plankton), which float in the sea, also capture carbon dioxide and make oxygen. In fact, the oxygen in every other breath you take comes from the oceans. That's why we have to protect our oceans and why increases in sea temperature from global warming is having a massive impact on these micro-organisms.

The carbon footprint of a vegan diet is less than half that of a meat eater's diet, so going vegan, or at least eating a largely plant-based diet, helps to reduce the impact we humans have on the planet.

Global warming might seem a big deal for us, but for the 800 million people on this planet who are undernourished, the biggest issue is simply getting enough food. It takes ten times as much land to grow grain, grass or soya to feed cattle in order to feed humans than to directly grow a source of protein, such as beans or lentils, and to eat those instead. The usual figure given is that you can *grow* ten times more protein on an acre than the protein you can generate raising beef on the same acre. However, one recent study estimates that a plant-based diet and associated agriculture can generate twenty times more protein than the equivalent piece of land needed for beef and twice that of eggs.[1]

If we all ate more plant-based foods, and distributed the food surplus, fewer people would need to suffer, or die, from being inadequately nourished.

Life and health is about balance

Maintaining the balance of life between oxygen (life) and oxidants (death) is your body's chief preoccupation. It does this with its own cellular recycling plants based on advance antioxidant systems. For this to work we need to take in a lot of antioxidants – vitamins C, E, the B vitamins, co-enzyme Q10, glutathione, alpha-lipoic acid, beta-carotene, anthocyanidins and resveratrol. A rich supply of these can be found in specific plant foods. In the next chapter I will explore how nutrients work together to keep you young, healthy and alive. That's another reason why moving in a plant-based-diet direction is a wise choice.

The increased intake in antioxidants from following a plant-based diet is one of the reasons for reduced disease risk in the vegetarian diet compared to meat eaters, but there are others, including the reduction in oxidants by not eating burnt animal fats. Let's look at the evidence for which kind of diet is associated with better health outcomes. There are very few major studies on vegans, as opposed to vegetarians, so I'll start by looking at what there is in relation to both, as well as studies relating to the level of vegetables and fruits eaten.

More fruit and veg means less premature death

Every study that I've ever seen shows that the more servings of fruit and vegetables a person eats the longer they live. Or rather, the less likely they are to die (from disease) during the duration of the surveys.

A classic study in this regard is a UK study that followed 65,000 people over the age of 35 over 7 years and found that those eating 7 or more servings of fruit and vegetables had a 42 per cent lower risk of death compared to those eating none.[2] As you can see in the chart below, the more servings of fruit and veg a person eats the lower the risk of dying prematurely. In this study fruit juice (devoid of fibre and high in sugars) and canned fruits (in sugary syrups) didn't reduce risk. It has to be the whole fruit.

How fruit and vegetable intake reduces risk of death

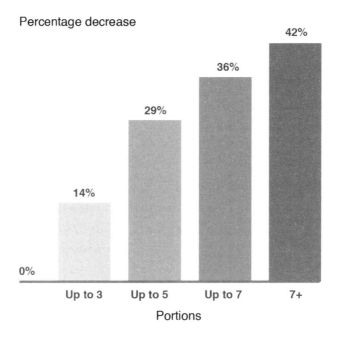

Based on data from Oyebode O, Gordon-Dseagu V, Walker A, et al., 'Fruit and vegetable consumption and all-cause, cancer and CVD mortality: analysis of Health Survey for England data', *Journal of Epidemiology and Community Health*, 2014;68:856–862.

Vegans have lower diabetes, heart disease and cancer risk

Almost every survey on vegans and vegetarians (and also pescatarians, who eat fish but do tend to have a more plant-based diet) shows a reduced risk of obesity, diabetes and heart disease, and their health statistics skew in the right direction, including the key one: living longer. Two recent reviews of all the evidence classified vegetarians a third to a half less likely to have diabetes than non-vegetarians[3] and another showed less cardiovascular disease[4]. A 2016 study reported that people who eat more animal protein rather than vegetable protein have a greater risk of diabetes. This large study followed over a hundred thousand people over several years, and found that over 15,000 of them went on to develop diabetes. The higher their intake of animal protein the greater was their risk of developing diabetes. For those in the top fifth for animal protein intake their risk went up by 13 per cent. According to the researchers, 'substituting 5 per cent of energy intake from vegetable protein for animal protein was associated with a 23 per cent reduced risk of diabetes'.[5]

A small study assigned 49 diabetics either a low-fat vegan diet or a conventional diabetes diet (which was low fat but not low carb, and contained meat), both of which were designed to be relatively low in calories. It found a significant extra decrease in HbA1c (a measure used to diagnose type-2 diabetes), lower levels of LDL (the so-called bad cholesterol) and total cholesterol, but no difference in weight loss between the two diets.[6]

Some of the clearest research regarding the benefits of a vegetarian diet has been done on Seventh-Day Adventists. At Loma Linda University, Dr Gary Fraser has been studying Seventh-Day Adventists in America, who live much longer than most people. Most, but not all, are vegetarian. Comparing Seventh-Day Adventists who did eat meat to those who didn't, his research showed that eating beef three times a week is associated with double the risk of heart disease – a difference of four to five years of life expectancy. Another study shows that vegetarian Seventh-Day Adventists have a reduced cancer risk of about one-third.[7]

What about vegans? Do they do better? In 2017 a meta-analysis pooling the results of all studies to date was conducted. 'This comprehensive meta-analysis reports a significant protective effect of a vegetarian diet versus the incidence and/or mortality from ischemic heart disease (–25 per cent) and incidence from total cancer (–8 per cent). A vegan diet conferred a significant reduced risk (–15 per cent) of incidence from total cancer.'[8] Another study looking specifically at breast cancer did not find a significant difference between vegetarians and non-vegetarians but did find that vegans had a 22 per cent lower risk compared to non-vegetarians.[9]

In some studies vegans are slightly ahead of lacto-ovo vegetarians (those who have milk and eggs) and those who include fish but, in other studies, pescatarians who also ate a high plant-based diet do best. It seems that eating healthy plant-based diets confers many benefits including decreased overall mortality, less heart disease and diabetes, and lower cholesterol, blood pressure, insulin, HbA1c and inflammation.[10] A vegan diet (which by its very nature excludes dairy products and eggs) seems to be best in terms of reduced cancer risk.

The dangers of meat and milk

Both meat and dairy are, of course, not a part of a vegan diet, but it's worth knowing the benefits of avoiding these foods.

The flip side of the positive message outlined above are the studies showing that high meat consumption, especially processed meat, but also red meat, is associated with worse health outcomes. Dairy products are associated with increased risk of prostate and breast cancer, as well as colorectal cancer.

Let's start by looking at what studies show us about meat consumption. All studies I have seen show that processed meat is much worse than red meat. According to Professor Walter Willett, from Harvard Medical School, large US-based studies show that the risks of death and disease from eating processed meats are several times worse than other meats, both red and white, and that eating 35g a day of processed meat (a serving every other day), is associated with a 20 per cent increased risk of premature death – mainly from cancer. The risk from processed meat starts to crank up with as little as 20g, half a serving, a day.

The very large European Prospective Investigation into Cancer (EPIC) study, which followed half a million people in 10 countries for more than 12 years, found that *moderate* meat consumption did not correlate with reduced life expectancy.[11] When the intake of red meat rose above 80g a day the risk of mortality slightly increased, whereas 160g or more significantly increased risk. White meat – chicken – made little difference, and, in fact, slightly reduced the risk of premature death. Both a large trial in the *Journal of the American Medical Association*[12] and the Holford 100% Health Survey on over 55,000 people, grade red meat as very slightly negative, while processed meat was right at the top of 'bad' foods, being as big a risk factor as sugary drinks. In our survey those eating meat two or fewer times a week, including none, had the greatest chance of being in optimal health, and those eating meat every day had the greatest chance of being in poor health. (This survey is available on the 100% Health Club website – see Resources.)

Meat fans may point out that these small percentage increases mean even smaller numbers of people actually getting cancer, or dying younger, but it is undeniable that all the evidence points in the same direction of too much meat, especially processed and red meat, being bad for you.

The problem with meat

Why is meat protein potentially bad for health? A meta-analysis of 30 studies clearly shows that measures of kidney function get worse at 25 per cent of calories or more of protein, which is the equivalent of eating meat three times a day.[13] Poor kidney function is common in people with diabetes. The negative effect on the kidneys seems to be mitigated by vegetarian protein, and although an excess of this could also be a problem, you'd have to eat a lot of tofu, quinoa and beans.

Another problem is the role of meat in raising insulin. Insulin-like growth factor (IGF-1) is a known cancer promoter, and insulin is something that you want to keep low. The higher your IGF-1 and insulin, the greater your cancer risk. Diets high in protein raise IGF-1.

A high-protein diet might also raise insulin because it is acid-forming. The more amino acids you eat, the more acid load your body has to deal with. The body can buffer short-term increases in acid load but consistently eating a high-protein diet results in the over-production of metabolic acids, which has been shown to impair insulin function and is associated with insulin resistance and reduced blood sugar control, as well as a higher incidence of diabetes.[14] Vegetable proteins, including beans and lentils, contain more of the alkaline minerals magnesium and potassium, and may be preferable in this regard.

Meat is also strongly linked to increased incidence of bowel (colorectal) cancer, which is the second most prevalent cancer in the UK. Each year more than 30,000 people are diagnosed with the disease, and around 18,000 die of it. Colorectal cancer is one of the fastest growing cancers, especially in younger adults. A plant-based lower carb and lower meat diet, and an active lifestyle, are conservatively estimated to be able to reduce the incidence of colorectal cancer by 60 per cent.[15]

Carcinogens in what we eat, exacerbated by putrefying food

(because of poor digestion and constipation) and microorganisms in an unhealthy gut, play a big part. The greatest risk factors are: eating a diet high in animal fats and processed and red meat (especially grilled, barbecued or burnt); a diet low in fibre; a history of polyps; smoking; excess alcohol; a lack of exercise; a lack of vegetables; a high calorie intake; and prolonged stress.

Grilling, burning and, especially, barbecuing meat produces known carcinogens called HCAs and PAHs, and processed and cured meat produce carcinogenic nitrosamines, a product of using nitrites in the curing process. Vitamin C, by the way, inhibits the formation of nitrosamines in the gut, so having a plant-based diet high in vitamin C, and/or supplementing it, helps to reduce risk. Meat also contains haem iron, found in red meat not white (it's what makes meat red), which is also a carcinogen.

Professor Martin Wiseman, World Cancer Research Fund International's Medical and Scientific Adviser says, 'The evidence on processed meat and cancer is clear-cut. The data show that no level of intake can confidently be associated with a lack of risk. Processed meats are often high in salt, which can also increase the risk of high blood pressure and cardiovascular disease.'[16] Other researchers report the same association.[17] The World Health Organization classifies processed meats, such as bacon, sausages and ham, as a carcinogen. Fish, on the other hand, is associated with a reduced risk of various cancers, and certainly no increase; however, fish and the essential fats that they contain can also be damaged by burning or barbecuing. The same is true for any vegan foods, especially fatty foods, that are burnt, browned or made crispy.

By eating a meat-free diet, substituting plant-based protein sources, which I'll explain in Chapter 5, you'll certainly be reducing your cancer risk.

Low carb diets, as we'll explore in Chapter 7, which have more protein from vegetable sources, do work well. An example of this was a study headed by Professor David Jenkins, who invented the glycemic index (GI – a measure of how much blood sugar rises after a certain food is eaten). He gave two groups of people a reduced-calorie diet: the first diet was low in 'slow carbs' (carbohydrates that release their sugar slowly) and high in fat and protein, but from vegetable sources not meat, while the second was higher in carbohydrates, and lower in fat and protein.[18] People in both groups lost nearly 4kg (8.8lb) in the four weeks, but those on the low-carb diet had greater reductions in their total cholesterol and LDL cholesterol levels. This diet was very close to my own low-GL diet, the principles of which are easy to follow on a vegan diet (more on this in Chapter 7).

The problem with milk

One of the best predictors of a country's rate of prostate cancer, and to a lesser extent breast cancer, is its milk consumption.[19] A landmark study found the highest risk of cancer death is in countries with the highest dairy consumption, such as Switzerland, Norway, Iceland and Sweden, with around 25 deaths per 100,000.[20] In stark contrast, in most Asian countries the risk is minimal, with deaths below 5 per 100,000 – in other words a fifth fewer deaths attributed to prostate cancer.[21] In such countries, where the diet consists mainly of whole grains, vegetables, fruits, tofu, soya milk and other soya products, and where milk is not a normal part of the diet, people are generally healthier, and breast and prostate cancers are much rarer than in the United States and Europe.

This is hardly surprising, since the evolutionary purpose of milk is to stimulate cell growth and to help the newborn infant to develop into a fully grown adult. All mammals stop consuming milk as soon as the initial growth phase is over, except for humans.

Milk helps cells to grow because it both contains the growth hormone IGF-1, and also stimulates the liver to produce more. On page 15, we saw how high levels of IGF-1 are strongly associated with an increased risk of cancer – 'a three- to fourfold increase in risk of breast, prostate or colorectal cancer' – as studied by Professor Jeff Holly from Bristol University. This opinion was confirmed in a Harvard University study of 20,000 men, which found that those with the highest levels of IGF-1 had more than four times the risk of developing prostate cancer than those with the lowest levels.[22]

There is a particularly strong link between dairy intake and prostate cancer. Indeed, according to the National Cancer Institute, all but four of 23 studies have found a positive association between the two.[23] A Harvard University study found that participants who consumed more than two dairy servings each day had a 34 per cent higher risk of developing prostate cancer than those who consumed few or no dairy products.[24]

The link with breast cancer is also well established, although not as strongly as for prostate cancer; however, it is increasingly being advised in many leading cancer treatment centres to avoid dairy products if you have breast cancer. The latest study finds that, while milk consumption increases risk, soya milk consumption reduces it. High-milk consumers had a 22 per cent increased risk whereas those who had substituted soya milk for dairy milk had a 32 per cent reduced risk.[25] Soya contains phytoestrogens, which reduce risk (see page 74 in Chapter 5).

The first study I know of started in 1937 in the UK, following a group of almost 5,000 children and recording their dietary habits. Sixty-five years later, an analysis of their reports revealed that those with a high dairy intake during childhood had three times the risk of developing colorectal cancer later in life.[26] Bladder cancer is also associated with high dairy consumption.

One of the prevailing myths is that you need dairy products for calcium to make stronger bones. Yet numerous studies have shown no increased bone density in children consuming more milk[27] nor in post-menopausal women consuming milk or supplementing calcium[28] and hence increasing their calcium intake. Certainly, we all need calcium (see Chapter 9) but taking in too much is not going to make your bones stronger. By far the biggest promoter of bone strength is vitamin D, which I talk about in Chapter 8.

Dairy products are not essential foods (obviously breast milk for an infant is a very different thing). For this reason, my diet has been dairy-free for the past 40 years.

The fibre factor

One of the potential problems of people who are not following a healthy balanced diet, whether they have a diet high in meat and dairy or are vegans and vegetarians who eat mostly processed foods, is getting enough fibre. A high-fibre diet shortens the time food takes to pass through the digestive tract and thereby reduces the exposure to carcinogens. This is especially true when eating what are known as soluble fibres, found, for example, in oats and chia seeds. We can minimise our risk of developing colorectal cancer by choosing a diet that is high in fibre. Unprocessed plants, especially when eaten raw, are naturally high in fibre. Most of the fibre in vegetables breaks down on cooking and therefore no longer assists digestion. Steamed vegetables retain more fibre benefit. You should be defecating with ease once, if not twice, a day. Few do, though, especially those on a high-meat diet. The Holford 100% Health survey of 59,000 people found that only two in ten people (17 per cent) have a satisfactory bowel movement every day, with 45 per cent straining.[29] These two symptoms combined suggest that close to half the adult population suffer from some degree of constipation. These symptoms are more prevalent in men, with only one in 10 having a satisfactory bowel movement daily.

Fibre helps to reduce the availability of carcinogenic compounds. Soluble fibre acts as fuel for the growth of friendly bacteria, which, in turn, lower the pH (and therefore raise the acidity) of the colon. Higher acidity in the colon is associated with a lower risk of developing colorectal cancer.

One study compared the faecal pH of South Asian vegetarian pre-menopausal women with that of Caucasian vegetarian and omnivorous women to see whether there was any link between this and their intakes of fibre, fat and cholesterol. The research found that there was indeed an association between high-fibre diets and faecal pH. It also showed that a vegetarian diet decreased the concentration of bile acids in faeces, a factor that has also been linked to a lowered chance of developing colorectal cancer.[30] The vegetarians also went to the loo more often. Another study found that a high-fat, low-fibre, high refined-carbohydrate diet also increases the activity of beta-glucuronidase, an enzyme secreted by toxic bacteria that can generate carcinogens in the colon.[31]

My conclusion, purely from a health point of view, is that a plant-based diet, avoiding (or greatly limiting) meat and dairy products, with plenty of vegetable proteins from nuts, seeds, beans and greens reduces a person's disease risk and extends healthy lifespan. But the key is to eat a lot of vegetables, as too much fruit and fruit juice, especially if you don't exercise much, can mean that you are consuming too much sugar. I go into this in more detail in Chapter 7.

Your quick guide to the benefits of a plant-based diet

- A plant-based or vegan diet is more carbon-friendly and would increase the amount of food that can be produced and hence feed more people, which becomes increasingly imperative as the population increases but the amount of farmable land stays the same.

- A largely plant-based or vegan diet is likely to extend your lifespan and reduce your risk of diabetes, heart disease and cancer, especially if you control your carbohydrate intake (see Chapter 7).
- Avoiding dairy products, a requisite for a vegan diet, is likely to reduce your risk of prostate, breast or colorectal cancer.

Chapter 3

Nutrients are Team Players

The science fiction of the 1960s envisaged a future in which humans would simply eat pills or powder containing the finite number of nutrients proved to be essential for the human machine to function. Yet, as each decade passes, we learn more and more about the complexities of the human body and nutrition. Of the 50 currently known essential nutrients, all interact with other nutrients and can be said to work in synergy. But there are many other factors in food, not classified as 'essential', that also help or hinder essential nutrients in their work.

Knowing this, it would be unrealistic to prescribe one nutrient for the treatment of disease. Indeed, in some circumstances prescribing one nutrient can exacerbate a deficiency in another, as you'll see in Chapter 9 on minerals. Iron, for example, is a zinc 'antagonist', thus making zinc deficiency worse. Both are frequently deficient in the diet. Prescribing excessive amounts of iron, for example in the case of anaemia, exacerbates an undiagnosed or untreated zinc deficiency. Since zinc is a critical nutrient for foetal development, this could have serious detrimental effects during pregnancy. Eating a wholefood diet, which provides both iron and zinc and many other nutrients, helps to ensure that there's no overt deficiency of just one nutrient.

Nutrients are synergistic

Some nutrients simply will not work without their synergistic mates; for example, vitamin B6, pyridoxine, is useless in the body until it is converted into pyridoxal-5-phosphate, a job done by a zinc- and magnesium-dependent enzyme. If a woman has premenstrual syndrome (PMS), for example, and is zinc or magnesium deficient, but takes only a vitamin B6 supplement because it has been recommended as helpful, it will not make any difference. Studies have shown that giving women zinc, magnesium *and* B6 relieves the symptoms of PMS much more effectively.

The vast majority of research in nutrition, however, has looked at the effects on health of a single nutrient. The results are not comparable with the effects of giving a person *optimum* nutrition: the right balance of all essential nutrients. For example, there is little evidence that individual vitamins or minerals can increase IQ scores in children; however, the combination of *all* vitamins and minerals, even if given only at RDA levels, has consistently been shown to produce a four- to five-point increase in children's IQ scores.[1] Similar combinations of vitamins, minerals and essential fats have produced massive reductions in the aggression of prison inmates, compared to placebo, in just two weeks.[2] These kinds of results are simply not seen with individual nutrients.

Understanding nutrients is essential for vegans

Why is this relevant to you as a vegan? Take B vitamins as an example. In Chapter 8 you'll learn that a family of B vitamins drive a fundamental process in the body and brain called 'methylation'. Methylation does just about everything, from helping to make hormones (such as insulin), neurotransmitters (such as adrenalin) and cells, especially brain cells, as well as switching genetic messages up and down (see epigenetics on page 15). Every two seconds there are a billion of these methylation reactions, which simply can't take place if you're deficient in either vitamin B6, folic acid or B12. Vitamin B3 also plays a minor part, as do magnesium and zinc. All of these are present in a wholefood diet – except B12. In Chapter 8 I explain why, as a vegan, you simply have to either supplement B12 or eat fortified foods supplemented with B12. If you don't, the other B vitamins can't do their job.

There are now hundreds of studies that show that the right nutrients in combination can produce improvements in health of a different league from that provided by individual nutrients. A classic example is the combination of B vitamins needed to lower homocysteine. This toxic protein in the blood tells you if your body is carrying out methylation properly. The higher your blood homocysteine, the less efficient your system is at methylation. It is an incredible predictor of disease risk, not only for cardiovascular disease but also for depression, Alzheimer's disease, miscarriage and the risk of birth defects, and many more conditions. It even predicts school performance! (I'll explain all this in Chapter 8 on vitamins.) Lowering homocysteine, and hence lowering your risk, is easy if you know how. You need an optimal intake of vitamins B6, B12 and folic acid, plus B2, zinc, magnesium and tri-methyl-glycine (TMG).

Few medical studies, however, have taken this on board. Most simply indicate that folic acid should be taken. This, by the way, is why folic acid is given during pregnancy – to lower homocysteine and reduce the risk of birth defects. Let's now take a look at what happens if you give one, two, three or all of these nutrients together. In a research study in Japan, patients with kidney disease, a condition strongly linked to high homocysteine, were divided into four groups: one group was given folic acid alone, another B12 alone, another folic acid and B12 together, and another folic acid, B12 and B6 together. The trial lasted for three weeks.[3]

Here were the results of this remarkable study:

Study into homocysteine and B vitamins

Supplement group homocysteine change	
Folic acid alone	17.3% reduction
B12 alone	18.7% reduction
Folic acid plus B12	57.4% reduction
Folate, B12 and B6	59.9% reduction

Notice that this extraordinary study revealed two very important principles:

1. The more nutrients provided, the greater the reduction in homocysteine.
2. The right combination of nutrients at the right dose can more than halve your homocysteine level, and your risk for homocysteine-related conditions, such as heart attack and stroke, in as little as three weeks!

Notice also that no group was given all the nutrients that lower homocysteine, including B2, zinc, magnesium and TMG. At the Institute for Optimum Nutrition we took six volunteers with raised homocysteine levels and gave them these nutrients. Their homocysteine levels dropped by 77 per cent – the combination was more than four times as effective as the conventional medical prescription of folic acid to lower homocysteine. That is the power of synergy and that is why the results provided by optimum nutrition are in a different league from those you read about in single-nutrient trials designed by those who think along the lines of a 'pill for an ill'.

Another example of this is provided by the interplay of anti-oxidant nutrients such as vitamins C, E, beta-carotene and others (including glutathione, co-enzyme Q10, lipoic acid and antho-cyanidins), which are found in good quantities in berries. They have some effect in isolation but are much more effective when they work together. They, like all nutrients, are team players.

How antioxidants work together

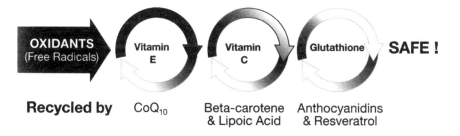

A free radical (see page 14), for example from a French fry/chip, is partially disarmed by vitamin E, further neutralised by vitamin C and finally by glutathione. Meanwhile the 'spent' glutathione gets reloaded by anthocyanidins, while vitamin C is reloaded by beta-carotene and lipoic acid, and vitamin E by CoQ10. These are the essential antioxidants working together as a team.

Antioxidants and the fight against harmful oxidants

In the illustration above you can see how nutrients work together. Free-oxidising radicals, sometimes called 'free radicals' or 'oxi-dants', are the bad guys produced from anything burnt, be it a cigarette, exhaust fumes or fried fat. The free radicals are like red-hot sparks that can damage your body. The antioxidants are like flameproof gloves that pass these hot potatoes along the line, gradually dissipating their potentially damaging properties. You need all of them to do the job properly and that's why I pay less attention to studies that just use one nutrient rather than multi-nutrient approaches.

This also emphasises why the place to start is a varied, whole-food and multi-coloured diet. If half your diet consists of beige foods, such as bread, pasta and pizza, you're just not going to get that healthy spread of antioxidant nutrients. Nature has actually colour-coded food for us. Different colours have different kinds of antioxidants and health-promoting polyphenols, compounds that also act as antioxidants (see page 48 for more on polyphenols); for example blue foods such as blueberries, blackcurrants, blackberries and elderberries are high in antho*cyan*idins (-cyan- means blue). These increase the powerful effects of a key antioxidant called glutathione, which is found in onions and garlic. Carrots and butternut squash – the orange vegetables – on the other hand, are high in beta-carotene, the 'vegan' form of vitamin A. The greener the foods, such as broccoli, spinach and kale, the more folate they contain. Rich colours – for example, from cacao and cinnamon – indicate other antioxidants and polyphenols. Cinnamon, for example, helps to stabilise blood sugar levels.

There are so many antioxidants and polyphenols that it all gets rather complicated. A simple measure of a food's ability to extinguish a harmful oxidant is called the oxygen radical absorption capacity (ORAC) and it gives you the food's overall antioxidant power. It's an objective measure of its ability to deal with the oxidant 'exhaust fumes' of life. Long-lived people tend to consume at least 6,000 ORACs a day, but what does this mean for your daily diet?

Each of the portions listed here equates to 2,000 ORACs, so any three each day will see you hitting that 6,000 target.

Portions containing 2,000 ORACs

⅓ tsp ground cinnamon	½ cup (75g/2¾oz) cherries or a shot of Cherry Active concentrate (see Resources)
½ tsp dried oregano	
½ tsp ground turmeric	1 orange or apple
1 heaped tsp mustard	½ pear, grapefruit or plum
8 pecan halves	⅓ medium avocado
¼ cup (4 tbsp) pistachio nuts	2 cups (120g/4¼oz) broccoli
7 walnut halves	½ cup (30g/1oz) red cabbage
1 cup (150g/5½oz) cooked kidney beans	1 medium artichoke or 8 spears of asparagus
½ cup (75g/2¾oz) cooked lentils	4 pieces of dark chocolate (70 per cent cocoa solids)
½ cup (60g/2⅛oz) blackcurrants, raspberries or strawberries	⅓ medium (150ml/5fl oz) glass red wine
⅕ cup (25g/1oz) blueberries	

Source: US Department of Agriculture

How to boost your antioxidant intake

In general, the most colourful and flavoursome foods have the highest antioxidant levels. Deep-coloured fruit, such as blueberries, raspberries and strawberries, also have high levels. For example, a single cup (125g/4½oz) of blueberries provides 9,697 ORACs. You would need to eat 11 bananas to get a similar benefit!

Therefore, not all portions of fruit and vegetables are equal. Both Day 1 and Day 2 in the following table contain the recommended 'five a day' but Day 2 has 8,000 more ORACs than Day 1.

A comparison of ORAC values in fruit and vegetables

Day 1		Day 2	
Fruit/vegetable portion	ORAC	Fruit/vegetable portion	ORAC
⅛ large cantaloupe melon	315	½ pear	2,617
1 kiwi fruit	802	½ cup (50g/1¾oz) strawberries	2,683
1 medium carrot (raw)	406	½ avocado	2,899
½ cup (60g/2⅛oz) peas (frozen)	432	1 cup (60g/2⅛oz) broccoli (raw)	1,226
1 cup (50g/1¾oz) spinach (raw)	455	4 asparagus spears (boiled)	986
Total	2,410	Total	10,411

I recommend not five but seven servings of fruit and veg a day. As an idea of how much that is, half a plate of veg in a main meal counts as two servings, so if you have some berries in your breakfast and a snack of fruit during the day, plus a carrot dipped in hummus for a snack, you've achieved seven portions of fruit and vegetables.

Polyphenol power

In recent years, a great deal of research has shown that a group of compounds known as polyphenols are just as important as a plant's antioxidant power, maybe even more so. They are a very broad group of compounds that plants produce to protect themselves from infection, UV radiation and other perils. We can benefit from these protective properties, too, because polyphenols seem to be able to switch off disease processes and switch on healthy genetic responses. Polyphenols are highly concentrated in many so-called superfoods, such as resveratrol in the skins of red grapes, isoflavones in beans, curcumin in turmeric, cinnamic acid in cinnamon and anthocyanidins in black elderberries and other berries.

It is possible to work out a general polyphenol rating for any food, in much the same way as we can calculate an antioxidant rating. Although such calculations are rather crude, they help us to identify the plants that pack the biggest health punch, especially as quite a few polyphenols also act as antioxidants; however, some do not: for example, peppermint is a terrific source of polyphenols but not so remarkable as an antioxidant, whereas basil is the opposite. I've listed some of my favourites below:

Polyphenol-rich foods

almonds	chia	parsley
apples	cinnamon	pecan nuts
artichoke	cloves	peppermint tea
asparagus	coffee	plums
avocado	curry powder	raspberries
basil	dark chocolate	red onion
beetroot	flax	red wine
black tea	ginger	rosemary
blackberries	green tea	sage
blackcurrants	kale	spinach
blueberries	lovage	star anise
broccoli	mint	strawberries
capers	olives	thyme
cherries	oregano	turmeric
chestnuts		

You'll notice that all these foods, as well as all the high-ORAC foods, are inherently vegan and natural. With the understanding that our complex adaptive system evolved in line with the natural world and the supply of largely fresh and organic foods, it becomes obvious that, rather than tampering with blunt man-made drugs, what we *eat* should be the cornerstone of health, and optimum nutrition should be a central part of resolving ill-health.

Your quick guide to eating 'teams' of nutrients for optimum health

The principle of synergy is a fundamental aspect of the optimum nutrition approach. Here are a few tips to bear in mind:

- There is no substitute for whole foods (unrefined and unprocessed foods). These contain hundreds of health-promoting substances, the importance of many of which we have yet to discover.
- Eat a varied diet, choosing from a wide range of different kinds of food.
- Do not supplement your diet with individual nutrients without also taking a good all-round multivitamin and mineral supplement (as I will explain in Chapter 11).
- Do not take a large amount of an individual B vitamin without also taking a B complex or a multivitamin.
- Do not supplement your diet with a large amount of an isolated antioxidant nutrient (such as vitamin C, E or beta-carotene) without also taking a good all-round multivitamin or antioxidant formula.

In the next chapter we'll explore the dark side: how modern living exposes us every day to thousands of anti-nutrients – pollutants, oxidants and hard-to-avoid chemicals – and why that is shaping the 21st-century pattern of diseases, from cancer to infections. This affects our understanding of what optimum nutrition means, as what we eat can provide the power to help the body detoxify from the unavoidable pollutants that we are all exposed to today.

Chapter 4

Anti-Nutrients – the Dark Side of Nutrition

Optimum nutrition is not just about what you eat – what you *do not* eat is equally important. Since the 1950s, over 3,500 man-made chemicals have found their way into manufactured food, along with pesticides, antibiotics and hormone residues from staple foods such as grains and meat. On top of that we have the negative health effects of genetically modified (GM) foods. Then there are oxidants from pollution, and ionising and non-ionising radiation from mobile phones, masts, smart meters and Wi-Fi routers. If you're taking medication, many medicines increase the demand for various nutrients. Most vaccines contain aluminium, which the body works hard to detoxify. On top of that are the toxins we choose to take in, be it from foods with chemical additives, cigarettes, alcohol, painkillers, or from the use of pesticides on non-organic foods that we eat. And then there are those that we create, for example, when curing or burning meat: PAHs, HCAs, nitrosamine and acrylamides, the carcinogen also found in many crispy snacks.

We also have air-borne pollution and particulates, radiation and microbes such as moulds, parasites and pathogenic bacteria. The bottom line is that mankind in the 21st century has a total load of anti-nutrients far in excess of those in our past – at what cost?

In the UK alone, we consume every year a staggering quarter of a million tons of food chemicals, 6 billion alcoholic drinks, 75 billion cigarettes, 80 million prescriptions for painkillers and 50 million prescriptions for antibiotics. In addition, 50,000 chemicals are released into the environment by industry and 400 million litres of pesticides and herbicides are sprayed onto food and pastures. Together, this constitutes a massive onslaught of man-made chemicals and pollutants, with undeniable global health and environmental repercussions.

Most of these chemicals are anti-nutrients. Anti-nutrients are defined as anything that interferes with the absorption or utilisation of a nutrient, or promotes its excretion. The more *anti-nutrients* you're exposed to, the more *nutrients* you will need. Each cigarette, for example, consumes vitamin C, thus smokers need much more vitamin C than non-smokers. The same is true of city dwellers exposed to more traffic pollution.

Dr Joe Pizzorno, in his books *The Toxin Solution* and *Clinical Environmental Medicine* (the latter co-authored with Walter J. Crinnion), makes a strong case that this exposure is a major driver of many of today's endemic diseases, including the stark increase in cancer. This is not an easy case to prove or practise science on, other than pointing out associations. What can be shown, however, is how over-exposure swamps the body's detox mechanisms.

Testing for anti-nutrients

Nutritional therapists (see Resources) might recommend testing for anti-nutrients if you're suffering with symptoms such as chronic fatigue, especially if you've had some sort of exposure to them, such as living next to a farm that sprays pesticides and herbicides, or you live in a particularly polluted environment.

Tests to check for anti-nutrients in the body are offered by 'functional medicine' laboratories, but you have to know what you're looking for. A useful first step used by nutritional therapists is a liver function test (included in Yorktest's Essential Healthcheck, see Resources). This tests two liver enzymes called AST and ALT, which have been shown to be pathologically raised due to exposure to a number of common anti-nutrients. ALT, for example, rises with increasing levels of PCBs (polychlorinated bisphenols), PAHs (polycyclic aromatic hydrocarbons) and heavy metals.[1] Another relevant test is homocysteine, which measures methylation, a critical detox mechanism in the liver. Homocysteine goes up with increasing exposure to a wide variety of anti-nutrients including heavy metals.[2]

Most people choose to become vegan partly for health reasons, and partly to protect animals from harmful and inhumane treatment. Consider then that you, too, are an animal and that your body also needs protection from this onslaught of anti-nutrients. While eating organic, avoiding single-use plastics and GM and refined foods, and drinking clean, filtered water are not an essential part of being vegan they do have the net effect of helping to protect the planet, animals and yourself.

Eat wholefoods and avoid refined foods

You might think that refined food that is free from artificial additives is OK, but it is not neutral. Whole food usually contains the nutrients needed by the body to process that food; for example, whole grains contain B vitamins, vitamin C, iron, zinc and magnesium, all needed by your body's metabolism to turn it into energy. If you eat refined white bread, pasta and cereals your body has to take those co-factor nutrients from its available supply.

Any food you eat that requires more nutrients for the body to make use of it than the food itself provides is effectively an anti-nutrient. Living on these foods gradually depletes the body of vital nutrients. In fact, two-thirds of the calories in the average person's diet in the Western world come from such foods. This means that a third of the diet needs to provide not only enough nutrients for general health but also enough to make up the deficit of nutrient-deficient food, and to combat other anti-nutrients such as vehicle pollution and pesticides.

Exactly what extra quantities of key nutrients we need to combat these anti-nutrients is not known, but it is certainly well in excess of the basic RDA/RNI levels. Take vitamin C, for example. How much vitamin C does a smoker need to consume every day to have the same blood level of vitamin C as a non-smoker, assuming that they both start with the same dietary intake equivalent to the RDA level? The answer is in excess of 200mg – roughly three times the RDA, according to research by Dr Gerald Schectman and colleagues at the Medical College of Wisconsin.[3] The same is true if you compare heavy drinkers with teetotallers. A heavy drinker needs to take in at least 500mg of vitamin C a day – six times the RDA – to have the same vitamin C blood level as a non-drinker. And what about pollution? If you live or work in an inner city, what is your need for antioxidant protection? Certainly it will be higher than the RDA and in the case of vitamin C, which detoxifies over 50 undesirable substances, including exhaust fumes, a daily intake of at least 1,000mg (1g) is more likely to be optimal. I've taken this into account when recommending optimal levels of nutrients in this book.

Toxic health problems

There are other assaults on our health that you might not have considered. We don't grow any GMO (genetically modified) foods in the UK, but it's possible we might be consuming them unwittingly from imported foods now or in the future. In 2009 the American Academy of Environmental Medicine (AAEM) publicly condemned GMOs in the food supply, saying that they posed 'a serious health risk'. 'Several animal studies,' according to their policy paper, reveal a long list of disorders, including: 'infertility, immune dysregulation, accelerated aging, dysregulation of genes associated with cholesterol synthesis, [faulty] insulin regulation, cell signalling, and protein formation, and changes in the liver, kidney, spleen and gastrointestinal system.' The policy concludes, 'There is more than a casual association between GM foods and adverse health effects.'

Glyphosate is one of the most widely used herbicides. It is classified as 'probably carcinogenic to humans' by the International Agency for Research on Cancer (IARC). You might use it in your garden and, if you don't, your neighbour might. Any food containing over 50 parts per billion of glyphosate cannot be called organic. In Italy the requirement for organic is below 10 parts per billion (ppb). My friend Bob Quinn, a farmer and campaigner for organic and chemical-free farming, has 8,000 acres of farms growing organic grain across Montana and neighbouring states. He is meticulous in avoiding the use of such pesticides and herbicides, yet even his grain has been measured with levels just over the 10ppb. The contamination is from rainwater. We are all exposed to glyphosates even if we choose to eat organic.

We are also exposed to PCBs, a non-biodegradable by-product of certain industries, even though these are now banned, and to increasing radiation from our Wi-Fi world.

The consequences of this are almost impossible to tease out. All we know is that human cells, in the 21st century, are under unprecedented assault. As we have seen, more than one in every three people now have a cancer diagnosis in their life. There are many other toxin-related health issues – such as chronic fatigue syndrome, or children with complex autistic/attention deficit-type issues, or adults with dementia (the youngest age of a diagnosis is now 23) – that are on the increase. Although it is known that a lack of B vitamins and omega-3 fats is driving dementia, certain drugs also have an effect: antacid drugs interfere with the body's ability to absorb B12, as does the diabetes drug metformin. These drugs are therefore classified as anti-nutrients – but what other anti-nutrients might be contributing to our mental decline? The conservative figure of deaths caused each year by pharmaceutical drugs, prescribed and taken in the correct doses, is 10,000,[4] although the true figure is likely to be much higher than this.

Increasing your detox potential

My personal choice has been to minimise my exposure to anti-nutrients as much as possible. The majority of the food I eat is organic. I avoid any GM foods. I have a plumbed-in water filter that purifies a number of anti-nutrients in the water I drink. I recycle as much as possible and generally minimise buying unre-cyclable products. I don't have a smart meter and have my Wi-Fi router quite some distance from where I sleep. I turn my mobile phone off at night and generally use the speaker for calls, thus not having it against my head. I have a landline with a corded phone (not a digital phone) for long chats. Fortunately, I don't need any medication. I don't smoke and I don't drink that much alcohol. These, of course, are personal choices made to generally decrease my total environmental load, which is a key part of the optimum nutrition equation (see 'The new model of health illustrated' on page 12). The other side of the equation is to support your body's detox potential.

Your body spends a lot of time and energy detoxifying. To put this in context, our metabolism either breaks things down, releasing the energy – for example, from carbohydrates – or it builds things up – for example, making proteins out of amino acids from food. Of all the maintenance work that takes place in the body two-thirds is spent detoxifying. Our bodies render many harmful chemicals harmless, and promote their excretion, by attaching them to a molecule that can export them out of the body. It's called 'conjugation'. It sounds like marriage but, in truth, it's more like handcuffing a criminal and either escorting them out of the building or putting them into jail, but in this case the harmful chemicals are put into storage in fat cells. That is why many overweight people, when they clean up their diet and start to burn off fat, experience symptoms of detoxification – feeling groggy, with headaches and various aches and pains.

Much of this detoxification happens in the liver, which needs large amounts of supportive detox nutrients to recycle and clear toxins from your body. Many of the antioxidant- and polyphenol-rich foods outlined in the previous chapter help the liver to detoxify, which is another reason to emphasise these foods in your diet. Detox diets, drinks and supplements with liver-support nutrients – such as glutathione and NAC in onions and garlic, curcumin from turmeric, anthocyanidins and polyphenols in berries, B vitamins, magnesium and potassium in greens – all help to support your body's detox potential.

Your quick guide to easing the anti-nutrient load

Here are some tips to help decrease the environmental load on your body:

- Invest in a good-quality, plumbed-in water filter and replace the cartridge every six months. Jug filters are also good, if you replace the cartridge as instructed.
- Buy organic. When not possible, wash or peel fruit and vegetables.
- Avoid GM foods.
- Never deep-fry foods, and switch to steam-frying (see page 239) instead of sautéing.
- Buy drinks in glass, not plastic, containers or cartons.
- Rearrange your daily schedule to minimise time spent in traffic.
- Drink alcohol very infrequently, and avoid smoky places.
- Avoid medical drugs unless they are the only viable option for treating a health problem. If you get frequent infections or aches, investigate the underlying cause rather than relying on painkillers or antibiotics.
- Reduce your exposure to Wi-Fi signals by using headphones or the speaker on your phone. Don't sleep near to your router or digital phone base station, and turn your mobile phone off at night.

Part 2

How Vegans Can Achieve Optimum Nutrition

To be a healthy vegan you need to get enough protein and essential fats, and avoid eating too many high-sugar carbohydrates. In addition, you need to focus on, and potentially supplement, the nutrients that are hard to get in sufficient quantities from plant-based foods alone: for example, vitamins B12 and D and the omega-3 fats EPA and DHA. This part explains what you need to know and do to be a healthy vegan.

Chapter 5

How to Get Enough Protein

It is a myth that you have to eat animals to get enough protein. Nor do you have to eat lots of extra protein to build muscle, if muscle building is your goal.

All proteins are made from a collection of 25 amino acids – the building blocks of the body; however, all 25 can be made from only eight *essential* amino acids (as shown in the diagram 'The amino acid family' overleaf). As well as being essential for growth and repair of body tissue, amino acids are used to make hormones, enzymes and antibodies required for immunity, as well as neurotransmitters (chemicals of communication) such as adrenalin and serotonin, which control your stress response and mood respectively.

Both the *quality* of the protein you eat, determined by the balance of these eight essential amino acids, and the *quantity* you eat, are important. If you are building a house, you need a certain amount of bricks, cement, wood and so on. Imagine each essential amino acid as one of these building components. If one is lacking, you can't build a house. Having foods, or food combinations, that provide close to the perfect balance of amino acids is important. A food that naturally contains all the eight essential amino acids is called a complete protein. Of course, animal protein is complete protein but, in turn, it was made from what the animal ate. A vegetarian animal, such as a sheep, derives all its protein from vegetable sources, such as grass. The same thing is true with fish through the food chain: a carnivorous fish, such as mackerel, eats a smaller fish, which ate a tiny organism called plankton, which derived its protein from algae or seaweed. Traced back in this way you can see that all protein ultimately derives from vegetable protein, which illustrates why vegetable protein is perfectly appropriate as a source of protein for everyone.

Let's start by examining which foods give you the best quality of protein before we look at how much you need, since the better the quality of protein the less quantity you will need. It's like building a house with less waste because you have everything you need and no more.

High-class proteins

The best foods to eat for protein are not necessarily those that are highest in protein to the *exclusion* of everything else. We don't just eat food to get one specific nutrient.

The pros and cons of a food's other nutritional constituents have to be taken into account to enable us to make an informed decision about the healthiest foods to eat. Comparing animal and vegetable sources of protein is interesting: for example, a lamb chop provides 25 per cent of total calories as protein and 75 per cent as fat, much of which is saturated fat. So even though it provides a lot of protein it also contains a lot of fat. Chia seeds provide only 18 per cent of total calories as protein, so they might be deemed a lesser source of protein, but what else do they provide?

The amino acid family

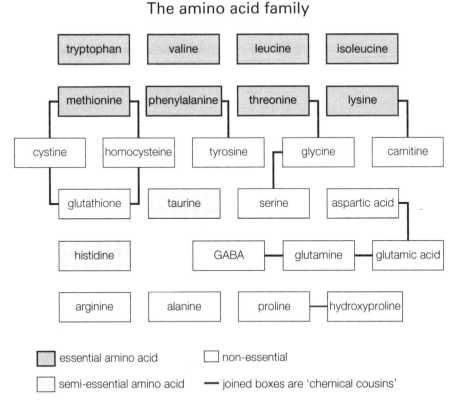

essential amino acid   □ non-essential

□ semi-essential amino acid   — joined boxes are 'chemical cousins'

For a protein food source to be classified as a complete protein it must contain the eight essential amino acids. These are found in meat, fish, eggs, soya and quinoa. The semi-essential amino acids are also found in these foods. Note that taurine appears to be essential in infancy.

Forty-seven per cent of the calories in chia are from fat, primarily polyunsaturated fats, and the remainder (35 per cent) are from slow-releasing carbohydrates (those carbs that release their sugar slowly, as I will explain in detail in Chapter 7). Also, although those carbs count towards the calories, much of it is in the form of insoluble fibre, which is the best kind of fibre, plus magnesium and other nutrients. So, chia seeds are a good all-round food. Half the calories in soya beans come from protein, so soya is actually a better source of protein than lamb, but its real advantage is that the remaining calories come from desirable slow-releasing carbohydrates.

How much of a food is protein determines how much you need to eat, but we'll get to the quantity issue in a minute. For now, let's focus on the balance of amino acids – the food's quality – which, if close to perfect, makes it a complete protein. (Please note that non-vegan sources of protein are included in the diagram below to give a comparison point. You might also find it useful to show to those who dispute the quality of vegan sources of protein.)

Protein quality and quantity

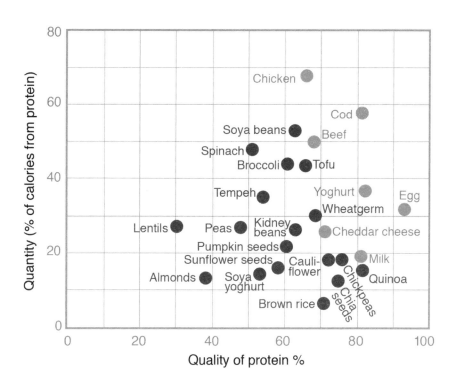

In the diagram opposite, along the horizontal axis, you'll see the quality of protein, with eggs scoring the highest percentage. In the plant world the best forms of protein are quinoa, tofu, brown rice, soya beans, seeds, nuts, peas and lentils. Although these are not all complete proteins individually, their protein profile can be increased through combining them with other foods, as I will explain. These foods are the cornerstones of vegan protein and therefore need to be present in your daily diet.

The reason lentils appear to be a low-quality protein is that they don't provide enough of the amino acids tryptophan and methionine. This means that 30g of the protein contained in lentils would provide only 10g of usable protein. That's like having bricks without enough cement. However, if you ate 30g of a combination of lentil protein and rice protein, the amino acid balance would be much better, giving 28g of usable protein. (You'd need a cup of each to achieve this amount of protein.) A visual demonstration of this is shown on the next page. Eggs, which provide the full complement of amino acids, provide a useful reference point.

You'll also see from the illustration on page 69 that combining foods from different food groups, such as vegetables with grains, grains with legumes (peas, beans and lentils) or legumes with nuts, helps to increase the quality of the protein. 'Flower' vegetables, such as the heads of broccoli and cauliflower, provide more usable protein than other vegetables, so eating a protein-rich vegetable such as these, or runner or broad beans or peas, with rice and lentils or beans is a great way to get enough good-quality protein.

Increasing the usability of protein

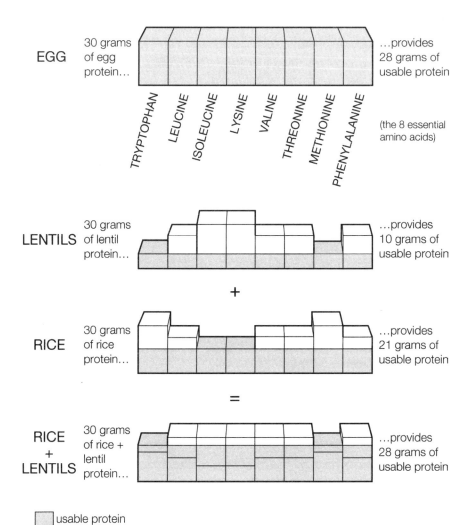

□ usable protein

Eggs contain adequate amounts of all the essential amino acids. By combining lentils and rice the same can be achieved with plant-based sources of protein.

How to combine plant-based sources of protein

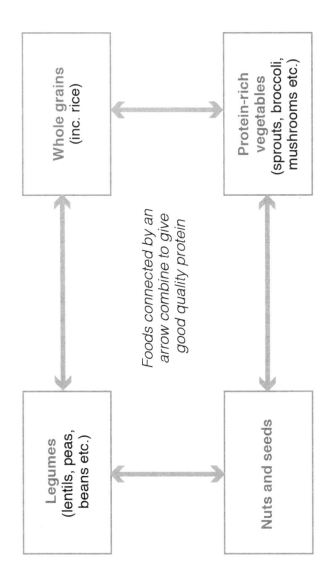

Whole grains (inc. rice)

Protein-rich vegetables (sprouts, broccoli, mushrooms etc.)

Foods connected by an arrow combine to give good quality protein

Legumes (lentils, peas, beans etc.)

Nuts and seeds

As you have seen, most protein sources are not complete, but they combine with other forms to create complete proteins. You don't have to be too pedantic about combining these food groups in every single meal, however. The body is always breaking down proteins, liberating amino acids into the bloodstream and providing a supply of amino acids to build new proteins. These are used to make new cells in the body, from muscle cells to brain cells, as well as forming hormones, and the brain's neurotransmitters, and enzymes – for example, enzymes to digest your food. You can think of the continuous supply of amino acids in the bloodstream like a builders' merchant: on hand to provide whatever your body needs to do its job. Your job is to top up this supply with what you eat, so eating a variety of food groups, as shown, over a 24- or 48-hour period is enough to ensure that you have sufficient quality of protein. A typical Indian meal, for example, combines lentils with rice, which would provide a good spread of all the amino acids. A traditional Chinese meal would do the same thing but using tofu and rice.

As a general principle, eat a varied diet with foods from each of these food groups.

How much protein do you need?

The government recommends that we obtain 15 per cent of our total calorie intake from protein, but gives little guidance as to the kind of protein. The average breast-fed baby receives 7 per cent of its total calories from protein and manages to double its birth weight in six months. This is partly because the protein in breast milk is of a very good quality and is easily absorbed. Assuming good-quality protein such as soya, quinoa, nuts or seeds, 10 per cent of calorie intake, or around 35g of protein a day, is an optimal intake for most adults, unless pregnant, recovering from surgery or undertaking large amounts of exercise or heavy manual work. (Note that this is the weight of protein and not the weight of the actual food. I provide weights for different foods on the next page.)

At most, we could say that 45g of protein a day provides more than enough, even to build muscle. That equates to 15 per cent of calories. (Protein has 4 calories per gram, so 45 × 4 = 180 calories. An average calorie requirement for a woman is 1,800 calories, so that's 10 per cent of calories; however, since the protein is unlikely to be perfect in its balance of amino acids – that is not 100 per cent complete – let's assume that it's 66.6 per cent usable, limited by its lowest amino acid. In that case, obtaining 15 per cent of your calories from protein would cover that.) There's a good case for increasing protein intake to this quantity, and to do some muscle-building resistance exercise, especially later in life, because maintaining muscle mass is key to good health. (The average person over 40 is losing 1 per cent, roughly 225g or half a pound, of muscle every year.)

In practical terms, if you aim for 15g of protein three times a day, or 25g twice a day, you'll have enough.

What does this mean in terms of the food you eat? All of the portions in the following table equate to 15g of protein. Don't eat more than three of these a day unless you're an endurance or strength athlete.

Food weights containing 15g of protein

Food	Weight	Serving (approx.)
Baked beans	310g (11oz)	¾ can
Black-eyed beans	175g (6oz)	⅓ can
Chia seeds	68g (2½oz)	½ cup
Chickpeas	164g (6oz)	1 cup
Hummus	200g (7oz)	1 small tub
Kidney beans	175g (6oz)	⅓ can
Lentils	165g (5¾oz)	⅓ can
Nuts (mixed)	100g (3½oz)	small packet
Peanuts	50g (1¾oz)	½ cup
Quinoa	125g (4½oz)	large serving bowl
Quorn	120g (4¼oz)	⅓ pack
Seeds (based on pumpkin)	50g (1¾oz)	½ cup
Soya milk	415ml (14½fl oz)	large glass
Soya mince	100g (3½oz)	3 tbsp
Tofu and tempeh	165g (5¾oz)	¾ packet

Is it dangerous to have more protein?

Getting more than a quarter (25 per cent) of your calories from protein might be harmful over the long term (although athletes both need and can tolerate more). The more protein you eat, the harder your kidneys have to work to eliminate nitrogen-rich waste products from your bloodstream. One meta-analysis of 30 studies found that kidney function declines significantly when consumption of protein exceeds 25 per cent of total calorific intake.[1] Poor kidney function is also a common symptom of diabetes. Getting too much protein should not be an issue on a vegan diet. (It certainly can be for those on a carnivorous diet. To put this into context, a cooked breakfast of sausage, eggs and bacon provides almost all the day's protein needs, so anyone who eats meat, fish and/or eggs three times a day will far exceed their limit.)

The two best sources of vegan protein, with a good balance of essential amino acids, which makes them of high quality, are soya and quinoa, so let's look at these foods, as they form a large part of many vegan diets.

Soya – good or bad?

Soya is a much-maligned food. It is blamed for the destruction of the rainforest, since large swathes of forest have been removed to grow it and a large proportion of it is used as the primary source of protein in all animal feed. Furthermore, much of the world's soya supply comes from genetically modified (GMO) soya, which has been altered to be resistant to herbicides. Genetic modification allows the biotech company to own the seed, or bean in this case, and also to supply the herbicide that kills the weeds but not the soya. None of this is the fault of the soya. By choosing non-GMO organic soya you are getting a very good source of protein.

The easiest way to eat soya is in the form of tofu, a curd made from the beans. There are many kinds of tofu: soft, hard, marinated, smoked and braised. Soft or silken tofu can be used to give a creamy texture to soups. Hard tofu can be cubed and used in vegetable stir-fries, stews and casseroles. Another soya product is tempeh, which is made from fermented soya beans. It has a much nuttier taste and a firmer texture than tofu. Since tofu is quite tasteless, it is best to marinate it or use it with well-flavoured foods or sauces. Natto is a Japanese source of protein derived from soya, but it is more mucilaginous and less palatable to the Western palate. Soya milk is also a good source of protein, with a 250ml (9fl oz) glass providing 8g of protein.

Soya, being high in phytoestrogens, has been mistakenly maligned because many people read 'oestrogen' and think of breast cancer. Plant-based phytoestrogens, found in most beans, including chickpeas (and the chickpea product, hummus), are actually good for you and help to protect against oestrogen-driven cancers. This is because the phytoestrogens effectively block the oestrogen receptors on cells, which means that fewer growth signals are sent to, for example, a breast cell. That is why communities who have a high intake of beans (and low dairy intake) have a lower rate of breast and prostate cancer.[2] The rural Chinese, who eat tofu and drink soya milk, but shun dairy products, have among the lowest incidence in the world of these cancers.

There is one slight concern regarding soya and this is its effect on the thyroid gland. The hormone thyroxine, which gives your body's energy metabolism a boost, is very slightly inhibited by a large intake of soya, or rather it could inhibit the absorption of the medication called l-thyroxine or synthetic thyroxine, that people who have an underactive thyroid are prescribed.[3] As a consequence they might need to take a little more. The effect is minor, and in healthy people who have sufficient iodine and vitamin C in their diet this is not an issue. (Iodine is required to make thyroxine, and vitamin C improves thyroxine levels – see Chapter 9.)

Quinoa

Grown in South America for 5,000 years, quinoa has a long-standing reputation as a source of strength for those working at high altitudes. It was the main protein source for the Aztecs.

Called the 'mother grain' because of its sustaining properties, it contains protein of a better quality than that of meat. Although known as a grain, quinoa is technically a seed. Like other seeds it's rich in essential fats, vitamins and minerals, providing almost four times as much calcium as wheat, plus extra iron, B vitamins and vitamin E. Quinoa is also low in fat: the majority of its oil is polyunsaturated, providing essential fatty acids. As such, quinoa is about as close to a perfect food as you can get. To cook it, rinse well, then add two parts water to one of quinoa, bring to the boil, then reduce the heat and simmer for 15 minutes.

Nuts and seeds

Chia seeds, and other seeds and nuts, are also an excellent source of protein. Each seed or nut also contains a wide variety of nutrients, because it is from these seeds that a strong tree or bush has to grow. This makes these foods an excellent and nourishing choice for vegans. Choose from chia, pumpkin and sunflower seeds, pine nuts, pecan nuts, pistachio nuts, peanuts, almonds, Brazil nuts, walnuts and hazelnuts.

Is vegan protein better for you than animal protein?

Almost every survey on vegans, vegetarians and pescatarians (a lot of studies look at all three) show a reduced risk of obesity, diabetes and heart disease, and their health statistics skew in the right direction, including the key one – living longer. Two recent reviews of all the evidence classify vegetarians a third to a half less likely to have diabetes than non-vegetarians[4] and another shows less cardiovascular disease.[5] But it is impossible to say that this is due to the protein element of their diet as such.

A survey in 2016, however, reported that people who eat more animal protein rather than vegetable protein have a greater risk of diabetes. In this large study of over 100,000 people, who were followed over several years, over 15,000 went on to develop diabetes. The higher their animal protein intake the greater was their risk of developing diabetes. For those in the top fifth for animal protein intake their risk went up by 13 per cent. According to the researchers, 'substituting 5 per cent of energy intake from vegetable protein for animal protein was associated with a 23 per cent reduced risk of diabetes'.[6]

In terms of actual 'intervention' studies, as opposed to surveys, the evidence follows the same direction. In a small study of 49 people with diabetes, participants were assigned either a low-fat vegan diet or a conventional diabetes diet (low fat, but not low carb, and including meat). Both diets were designed to be relatively low in calories. The study found significant extra decrease in HbA1c, the best measure of long-term glucose control, in the group following the vegan diet, as well lower LDL and total cholesterol, but no difference in weight loss.

As the Netflix film *The Game Changers* showed, there are plenty of body builders and top athletes who have all the muscle you could ever want, and enjoy good health and performance, while eating a plant-based diet. It is certainly sufficient, if not preferable.

Your quick protein guide

To make sure you're getting enough protein:

- Eat a portion (120–180g/4¼–6¼oz) of beans, lentils, quinoa, tofu, tempeh or natto every day. Combine incomplete proteins – for example, beans with rice – to make a complete protein.

- Eat a very large serving of vegetable protein in the form of broccoli, cauliflower, spinach, runner beans or peas every day.
- Eat a small handful of nuts or seeds – such as chia, pumpkin or sunflower seeds, pine nuts, pecan nuts, pistachio nuts, peanuts, almonds, Brazil nuts, walnuts or hazelnuts – as a snack most days.
- Have a glass of a nut or bean milk a day.

Chapter 6

The Importance of 'Brain' Fats

F ats are an important part of a vegan diet (any diet, in fact). They were unfairly demonised for many years, starting in the 1980s, which led to an increase in carbohydrate consumption, but two fats in particular are vital for your health. These are the two known essential fats – omega-3 and omega-6. They are essential because the body can't manufacture them, so they have to be provided via food or supplements. Omega-3 and -6 are especially important for the brain and nervous system, and therefore your mental health.

Omega-3 and -6 fats

The main sources of omega-3 fats are certain foods that grow in a cold climate, including walnuts, flax and chia seeds, but also leafy greens, seaweed and algae; and oily fish. The main plant source of omega-6 fats is seeds, especially those grown in a hot climate. Sunflower and sesame seeds, and their oils, are a good example.

The omega-3 and omega-6 fat family tree

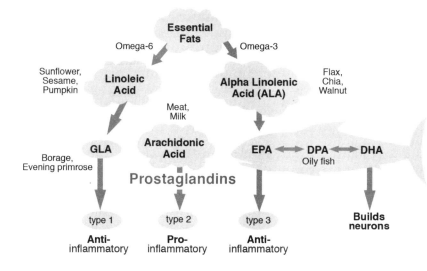

If you look at the diagram above you can see that the fats at the top progress into different forms at the centre – these are the types of oils that are most beneficial to the body.

In the case of the omega-6 fats, GLA (gamma linolenic acid), for example, is more biologically active than linoleic acid above it, making prostaglandins that, among other things, help to balance hormones and control inflammation. However, if we take sunflower oil as an example, it is mainly comprised of linoleic acid, which makes up 60 per cent of its fats. It provides only 0.1 per cent of GLA, so the body has to *convert* the linoleic acid into GLA. In contrast, borage oil and evening primrose oil are potent sources of GLA: borage oil is 22 per cent GLA and evening primrose oil is 10 per cent GLA. (Note that GLA can also be turned into the omega-6 fat arachidonic acid, which is found in meat and dairy products, but although it is essential you don't want too much arachidonic acid because it encourages inflammation by making type-2 prostaglandins.)

On the right-hand side of the diagram you can see the omega-3 fats. These start off as alpha linolenic acid (ALA), and need to be processed by the body into EPA and then DHA, which are the more active forms of omega-3. EPA is a potent anti-inflammatory, as well as an effective anti-depressant, and protects against heart disease, while DHA is a vital structural fat that builds neurons and hence the brain and the eyes; it is therefore linked to mental health and visual acuity. Very little ALA in plants can be converted into DHA: the conversion varies from 0.05 per cent up to a maximum of 6 per cent (see page 83).

Both EPA and DHA are the most concentrated in oily fish – these are fish such as salmon and mackerel that eat smaller fish – and their oils. Cod liver oil is also a direct source; however, DHA can also be derived from seaweed, and vegan supplements of DHA are available, some also providing EPA made by concentrating the DHA present in the oils of algae or seaweed.

Getting enough omega-6 and ALA from a vegan diet

If you eat nuts, seeds and leafy greens, and ideally some seaweed, you can certainly get enough omega-6 and enough of the omega-3 ALA on a vegan diet; however, this is something you need to have in your mind's eye when choosing which foods to eat.

An easy way to increase the amount of seaweed in your diet is to eat, for example, dried nori seaweed in the form of a snack (see Resources, page 261, for some suggestions), and add it to salads as a garnish. Also, I suggest that you favour the nuts and seeds higher in omega-3 fats than those higher in omega-6, because these two families of fats compete to some extent. If you have too much omega-6 in your diet, which is common, this can make a shortfall in omega-3 worse. Omega-3 deficiency is much more common than omega-6 deficiency.

In practical terms this means eating daily:

- A small handful, or a heaped tablespoon, of walnuts, pecan nuts, flax seeds, chia seeds, hemp seeds and/or their oil. (Pumpkin seeds contain both omega-3 and -6 and are the next best thing. Sunflower and sesame seeds are higher in omega-6, so don't go overboard on these.)
- One or two servings of dark green, leafy veg – especially those that grow in colder climates such as kale, broccoli, Brussels sprouts – or a serving of seaweed such as nori.

When using oils in cold food, such as salad dressings, you could also use flax, walnut or hemp seed oil. Chia oil is also delicious but is not widely available.

Fats for cooking

It is preferable not to fry, and especially deep-fry, too often. The reason for this is that high temperatures damage the essential fats and create harmful oxidants once the oil has passed its smoke point. When using oils for cooking, one of the oils with the highest omega-3 to omega-6 ratio, and with the highest smoke point, is rapeseed (but make sure you use a virgin, often called cold-pressed, oil). Sunflower oil, in contrast, provides only omega-6. You could also use an almost saturated (mono-unsaturated) fat, with a high smoke point, such as coconut oil, or olive oil. Saturated fats are solid at room temperature, which is why olive oil can go hard in the fridge.

DHA – vital for the brain and for the growing child

The guidelines on the previous page will give you enough of the omega-3 ALA. The problem is that the conversion of ALA into EPA, and especially into DHA, which is critical for the brain, is very little, as we saw on page 80. You'd have to eat a small mountain of flax seeds, or quantities of flax oil, to bump up your DHA level a little. DHA makes up over 90 per cent of the structural fat in the brain, so it's absolutely vital, not only for brain function, but also for brain development during pregnancy and early childhood. DHA is also strongly linked to reducing the risk of dementia later in life, thus protecting the brain from degeneration.

There is a compelling argument that we became human, despite sharing essentially the same genes as chimpanzees, because our hominid ancestors ate a marine-food diet, which would have been instrumental in building our bigger brains.

DHA is essential if you're pregnant or planning a pregnancy. It builds the baby's brain, and maintains your own, but the foetus will rob your stores of DHA and therefore your brain, while it builds its own – if there is an insufficient supply in your diet. Babies whose mothers supplement with DHA have increased brain size.[1] An infant also needs a healthy supply of DHA in early life, and in breast milk. There is extremely compelling evidence that vegans need to supplement DHA both in preparation for, and during, pregnancy and breast-feeding, as a lack of DHA is very common on a vegan diet and is strongly linked to pre-term babies, as well as decreased cognitive development and an increased risk of anxiety and depression in the mother. The evidence for this is discussed later in this chapter, on page 86. Fortunately, vegan DHA supplements derived from algae or seaweed are now available – and they work. A review of studies concludes that 'algal sources of DHA significantly improve [blood] DHA concentrations.'[2]

Vegetarians and vegans have, on average, less than half as much

EPA and DHA in their blood than those who eat fish; for example, a small study in Finland compared blood levels of Finnish vegans and non-vegetarians. Although they found higher levels of total omega-3, mainly from ALA, in the vegans, they found significantly lower levels of EPA (0.63 vs 2.33) and DHA (0.85 vs 2.25) in the vegans versus the non-vegetarians.[3]

While the general view is that only about 5 per cent of ALA is converted into EPA (studies have reported from 0.2 per cent up to 20 per cent), thereby demoting the value of vegetable sources of omega-3, even less is converted to DHA. The Flax Council reported 'most studies showing a conversion rate of about 0.05 per cent[4], although one study reported a figure of 4 per cent.'[5] Either way, not much gets converted. Younger women, it appears, convert more.

A major study carried out by Dr Ailsa Welch and colleagues, from the School of Medicine Health Policy and Practice at the University of East Anglia, rigorously analysed the omega-3 intake in the diets of more than 14,000 people in Norfolk.[6] Blood plasma levels of EPA and DHA were also assessed in a third of participants to work out how much actually gets through from the diet. One interesting finding was that dark green leafy vegetables also provided a significant portion of omega-3s (as does meat among meat eaters), but not nearly as much as oily fish.

The body can convert vegetable sources of ALA

Dr Welch's study showed that, as you would expect, the more fish – especially oily fish – eaten, the higher the blood plasma levels of EPA and DHA, with supplement takers having very high levels. However, what was particularly interesting was that the *difference* in circulating levels between non-fish-eating vegetarians, including vegans, and fish-eaters was not nearly as great as might be predicted. This was especially true in women. The implication is that when you are deprived of a direct source of EPA and DHA, the body might convert more from vegetable sources of ALA. Another possible reason why younger women might convert vegetarian sources of ALA more effectively is that oestrogen might help the process. This would make sense from an evolutionary perspective since it is in pregnancy that these essential fats are most important. Even so, are vegetarian sources of omega-3 sufficient? I asked Dr Welch. 'Until we know more about enriched sources of ALA – such as flax seeds, walnut, walnut oils, leafy, dark green vegetables – we should still be cautious as to whether you can really get enough without fish', she told me. In my opinion any vegan, but especially a pregnant vegan, is wise to supplement a vegan source of DHA derived from seaweed.

Does plant-based omega-3 (ALA) keep you healthy?

The above study didn't look at the health implications as such, but there is growing evidence that having a high intake of omega-3 ALA, from greens, nuts, seeds and their oils, has positive benefits. A survey of Eastern European countries found that the higher the intake of ALA, the lower the risk of cardiovascular disease[7], as did another survey in Costa Rica[8]; however, studies where ALA was given versus fish oils have *not* shown cardio-protective effects – as in fewer heart attacks or cases of high blood pressure – nor any significant conversion to DHA. Japan has among the highest levels of fish consumption and very low disease rates; in the UK, and with most other developed Western societies, it's the reverse. So the investigation into the benefits of fish oils compared to vegan versions of ALA continue; however, there is another aspect of omega-3 oils to consider.

One of the measures of cardio-protection is a high heart-rate variability (HRV). A high intake of omega-3 is both associated with high HRV and a low risk of cardiac death. A recent study in the *British Journal of Nutrition* compared vegans and omnivores and reported a lower HRV in vegans.[9] Whether or not this translates into less cardio-protection remains to be seen.

Omega-3 in pregnancy – why DHA supplementation is essential

Earlier we saw how important DHA is for pregnant women and during breast-feeding. A lack of this is so destructive that supplementing is essential. As we have seen, a conversion to DHA is especially important in pregnancy to build the baby's brain, but it's also important for the mother. The most compelling case for ensuring you achieve enough DHA comes from studies that clearly indicate low levels of omega-3 DHA predicts the risk of pre-term babies, who are more likely to have developmental problems. Furthermore, a lack of DHA early in pregnancy appears to have knock-on effects, even eight years later, on children's cognition. Given that the woman's ova takes a month to grow to be ready for pregnancy, and then starts the rapid cell division of foetal growth once fertilised, achieving good nutrition pre-conceptually, and certainly from the start of a pregnancy, is very important. As DHA is an oil, it's usually excluded from prenatal multivitamins. There is a powder form that is used in some supplements, but it is only one-third DHA, and therefore doesn't provide an adequate enough supply.

Professor Michael Crawford and colleagues, from the Institute of Brain Chemistry at the Chelsea and Westminster Hospital, have found that when there is a lack of DHA the foetal brain substitutes a type of oleic acid as a replacement structural fat, and high levels of this fat, with low levels of DHA, in the blood of pregnant mothers predicts the risk of pre-term babies most accurately.[10] Other studies have shown similar risks; for example, a Danish study found that those pregnant women with the lowest levels of EPA plus DHA in their blood, comparing the lowest fifth to the highest fifth, had ten times the risk of a pre-term baby.[11] Those in the lowest third for DHA levels had approximately three times the risk. A Norwegian study showed that supplementing omega-3 from fish oil during pregnancy resulted in both longer (fewer pre-term) pregnancies and bigger babies.[12] Another study found that higher DHA has also been linked to taller infants, both at birth and 12 months and five years.[13] Babies whose mothers supplement with DHA have increased brain size.[14]

Meanwhile, a substantial ongoing study of women and their children in the Avon area measured the fish intakes of women while pregnant and the subsequent development of their children.[15] Following analysis, the recommendations stated that 'consumption of less than 340g/week (three servings of fish a week) in pregnancy was detrimental, that is, increased the risks for low verbal IQ and abnormal behaviours among children'. The Avon study has also shown that maternal omega-3 intake from seafood predicts the level of 'acting before thinking' in children eight years later. As a vegan you won't be eating fish, but this does illustrate why it's vital for vegans to supplement the kind of amount that you'd get from three servings of fish a week.

Not all studies, however, have proven positive effects for DHA on children's intelligence. A study giving 800mg of DHA in the last third of pregnancy found no improved intellectual abilities in children seven years later.[16] It is possible that this study gave DHA too late in the pregnancy, or for too short a time, since brain development is most rapid early on.

The Avon study has also found that the intake of seafood, thus EPA and DHA, also predicts the mental health of the pregnant woman. They found that vegetarian women or those eating no fish were more likely to have high levels of anxiety than those obtaining 1.5g of omega-3 – roughly three servings of fish – a week.[17] This illustrates how these omega-3 fats are important, both for the brain and the nervous system.

The overall benefit of ensuring enough DHA in pregnancy, whether from fish, or supplements of purified fish oils (which are therefore mercury free), or algal-derived DHA, is certainly compelling and a message that needs spreading as more and more women turn vegan. See below for suggested optimal levels.

Supplementing EPA and DHA

As a vegan, the wise precaution is to supplement EPA and, most importantly, DHA derived from algae or seaweed. The basic recommendation for all is to achieve an intake of 250mg of combined EPA and DHA. This serves as a good guideline for supplementation, given the rather low conversion of ALA into EPA and DHA. Most vegan DHA supplements provide around 150–250mg plus 80mg of EPA, so about 250–300mg in combination. Time will tell what an optimal intake for brain function will be, but there is a good case to double this to 500–600mg of combined EPA plus DHA during pregnancy and perhaps later in life, to reduce dementia risk, as well as eating omega-3-rich plant-based foods. This is what I take.

An ideal level of DHA alone during pregnancy is 250–300mg a day. This is equivalent to what you'd get from two servings of oily fish, or three servings of fish, a week. Most vegan DHA supplements provide about 150–250mg so you'll need at least one of a high-potency product and two if it is not so concentrated. Fish oil omega-3 supplements usually provide 300mg per capsule, which is an option for less strict vegans.

Phospholipids and choline

Neurons – brain and nerve cells – are primarily made out of what is called 'phosphorylated DHA'. This is DHA that is bound to a kind of fat called a phospholipid.

Seafood contains phosphorylated DHA, but DHA supplements, whether derived from fish oil or algae, are not phosphorylated. Hence, the DHA from a supplement needs to be attached to phospholipids to work. This attachment is done by a process using B vitamins, called methylation. It's a bit like using those glues where you have two tubes and have to mix a squeeze of one with the other for the glue to work. The 'mixer' in this case is the B vitamins in your body attaching the DHA to the phospholipids. If you have no phospholipids, or no DHA or B vitamins, the mix is not going to work. You'll learn more about this in Chapter 8 on Vitamin Essentials, because vitamin B12, another nutrient that vegans need to supplement, is vital for healthy methylation.

Phospholipids

There are several different kinds of phospholipids with strange names all starting with 'phosphatidyl', such as phosphatidylcholine, phosphatidylserine, phosphatidylinositol and phosphatidylethanolamine. To a large extent these can all be made from phosphatidylcholine. As a group of nutrients they are classified as semi-essential because we can make some, but not enough for optimal health and especially optimal brain health.

As a consequence, there are moves afoot to classify choline (which can be easily attached to the 'phosphatidyl' part) as an essential nutrient with a recommended intake. This has come about due to the growing evidence that insufficient choline in pregnancy leads to cognitive impairment and developmental delay. This is particularly important for vegans because, like DHA, there's not so much choline in plant-based foods, but there is some in foods such as quinoa, soya, beans, nuts and broccoli – which are also important foods for protein, as we saw earlier.

Choline

Currently, an adequate intake of choline is defined as between 400mg and 520mg a day, the latter amount for pregnant and breast-feeding women. This is based on how much choline you need for healthy fat metabolism, liver function and reducing homocysteine levels (see pages 43–44 for more on this). You also need choline to utilise cholesterol in the liver and brain. Cholesterol is a vital brain component, but it has to be contained between the phosphorylated DHA. It's like a sandwich. But these levels don't take into account what's being learnt about choline's role in brain development.[18] A good estimate of optimum daily choline intake would be at least 500mg and you could perhaps double this in pregnancy. Choline is not included in most prenatal supplements, so this is something you'll need to either include in your diet or supplement (see below).

Most important is choline's role in building, and maintaining, a healthy brain. A pregnant woman's intake plays an important role in shaping the cognitive abilities of her child. Twenty years ago we knew that pregnant rats fed choline halfway through their pregnancy had more connections between brain cells, plus improved learning ability and better memory recall.[19] Now we know that it's true for babies, with several recent trials showing similar results, indicating that more choline in pregnancy enhances cognitive development.

An example of this is a study where women in their third trimester of pregnancy were given either 480mg of choline or almost double this – 930mg. The babies' information processing speed was then tested at 4, 7, 10 and 13 months. Not only were the babies of the mothers who were given the higher dose faster but also the longer the mother had been given even the lower dose, the faster were the child's reactions. The authors concluded that 'even modest increases in maternal choline intake during pregnancy may produce cognitive benefits for offspring'.[20] Seven years later, there were still memory advantages in the children whose mothers had extra choline during pregnancy.[21]

Babies are born with blood choline levels three times higher than their mother, illustrating how vital this nutrient is for building neuronal connections, which newborn babies do at a rate of up to a million new connections a second! An optimal intake for brain function is likely to be a lot higher than the 400–500mg recommended for adults, and higher still in pregnancy.

Brain cells are made of a membrane containing choline (and other phospholipids) attached to the omega-3 fat DHA. Without choline, therefore, the omega-3 doesn't work. The attaching of the two depends on methylation, a process that is dependent on B vitamins, especially B12, folate and B6. Choline helps methylation, and healthy methylation, indicated by a low blood level of homocysteine, helps to synthesise choline. You need all three – DHA, choline and B vitamins, especially B12 – so if you are lacking in DHA, or in vitamin B12, then you'll be doubly dependent on getting enough choline.

Choline-rich foods

Although the richest dietary sources of choline are fish, eggs and organ meats, there is a significant amount of choline in plant-based foods as well, notably: soya, as in tofu and soya milk; quinoa; seeds, including flax seeds; nuts such as almonds; peanuts; and cruciferous vegetables such as broccoli, cauliflower and Brussels sprouts.

On the face of it, it does appear that vegans, especially those planning pregnancy, need to become choline-focused in relation to choosing the most nutritious daily foods, and possibly also supplementing, but there is not yet conclusive evidence showing that vegan mothers are at risk, because that specific research hasn't been done. However, it is likely that they are because their diet is often lacking in this nutrient. One of the insights that has come out of studies on omega-3 DHA is that vegan mothers might convert more vegan omega-3 ALA into DHA as an evolutionary imperative, as we saw earlier – not that a top-up with supplementation isn't still the recommendation, however. Could it be that vegan mothers make more choline if needed, since it is so important for brain development? There are too few studies involving vegans to know the definitive answer to this question.

One recent study, however, looked at choline levels in the breast milk of vegans, versus vegetarians and non-vegetarians. There was no significant difference, and the author of the study concluded, 'This suggests that maternal plant-based diet by itself is not a risk factor for low breast-milk choline.'

The vegan community is certainly divided on this issue. Of course, the safe or cautious position to take, while the science unravels, is to supplement choline during pregnancy.

But what intake of choline can you achieve from a vegan diet alone? Here's a list of the best plant-based foods for choline, listed in the order of how much you could get in a reasonable serving.

Choline quantities in foods*

Food	Choline per serving	Per 100g
Soya milk (1 cup/ 250ml/9fl oz)	57mg	23mg
Shiitake mushrooms (1 cup/145g/5oz)	54mg	37mg
Soya flour (12.5g/½oz)	24mg	192mg
Peas (1 cup/ 160g/5¾oz)	47mg	30mg
Quinoa, raw (⅓ cup/ 60g/2⅛oz)	42mg	70mg
Beans, raw (⅓ cup/ 60g/2⅛oz) black, white, pinto, kidney	40mg	67mg
Broccoli, cauliflower or sprouts (1 cup/ 90g/3¼oz)	36mg	40mg
Tofu (½ cup/ 125g/4½oz)	35mg	28mg
Hummus (½ cup/ 1 20g/4¼oz)	34mg	28mg
Chickpeas (¼ can)	33mg	33mg
Baked beans (¼ can)	31mg	31mg
Flaxseeds (small handful)	22mg	78mg

Food	Choline per serving	Per 100g
Pistachio nuts (small handful)	20mg	71mg
Pine nuts (small handful)	18mg	65mg
Cashews (small handful)	17mg	61mg
Wholegrain bread (2 slices/50g/1¾oz)	17mg	34mg
Avocado (½)	14mg	28mg
Almonds (small handful/50g/1¾oz)	12mg	42mg
Peanuts (small handful)	12mg	42mg
Wheatgerm (tbsp 7g/¼oz)	12mg	178mg
Almond or peanut butter (tbsp)	10mg	61mg

Source: USDA choline content database and https://nutritiondata.self.com

* Many foods have not been analysed for choline, and measurements do vary, so this is a guide rather than a definitive list.

What does this mean for your daily diet? Here are some vegan foods that you could include in your meals to maximise choline intake, and how much each food would give you (I'm not including all foods that you would eat at these meals, just those ingredients that deliver a significant amount of choline):

Food	Choline
BREAKFAST	
A cup of soya milk (250ml/9fl oz)	57mg
Small handful of nuts or seeds (flax, chia, almonds, etc.)	20mg
LUNCH	
A cup of cooked quinoa (⅓ cup/55g/2oz raw)	43mg
A serving (100g/3½oz) of either broccoli, cauliflower or Brussels sprouts	36mg
½ avocado	14mg
SNACKS	
A tbsp of almond or peanut butter	10mg
Hummus (½ cup/120g/4¼oz)	34mg
2 slices of wholegrain bread	17mg
DINNER	
A serving of tofu (125g/4½oz) or beans	35–40mg
Shiitake mushrooms (½ cup/35g/1¼oz)	27mg
A serving (100g/3½oz) of either broccoli, cauliflower or Brussels sprouts	36mg
Total	**332mg**

The recipes in Part 3 that are choline friendly are: Wild Mushrooms on Toast; Butternut Squash and Tenderstem Broccoli Salad; Peruvian Quinoa Salad; Chestnut and Butter Bean Soup; Broccoli Soup; Beetroot and Borlotti Bean Soup; Chickpea, Carrot and Coriander Soup; Sun-Blush Tomato and Black Olive Chickpea Salad; Roasted Chickpea and Lemon Tabbouleh; Cauliflower Dhal; Teriyaki Tofu; Bean and Mushroom Bolognese; Quinoa Pilaf with Red Pepper and Pumpkin Seeds; Tofu Noodle Stir-Fry; Baked Falafel; Puy Lentils with Porcini Mushrooms and Thyme; and Quinoa Salad with Olives, Tomatoes and Pine Nuts.

In reality you are unlikely to achieve the 332mg total listed in the table above every day, and it would be quite limiting on your food choices, so a realistic target would be to achieve 300mg of choline from food. If you are aiming to achieve 500mg, which is the low end of optimal – more than this might be optimal in pregnancy – that leaves a shortfall of around 200mg of choline, suggesting the need for supplementation.

The most direct source of choline is from soya-derived lecithin granules and capsules. A flat tablespoon of lecithin granules (7.5g), which has a neutral and pleasant taste and can be sprinkled on cereals, in shakes and soups or eaten as it is, provides 1,500mg of phosphatidylcholine and around 200mg (13 per cent) of choline. Some 'high phosphatidylcholine' lecithin, sometimes called 'high PC lecithin', is 18 per cent choline, thus you need less – approximately a flat dessertspoon (2 teaspoons).

One tablespoon of lecithin granules equals three 1,200mg lecithin capsules (if taking 'high PC', two capsules would suffice). I suggest that this is a sensible addition to a completely vegan diet. (If your diet is plant-based most, but not all, of the time, the addition of two eggs, or an egg and a fish serving, would achieve 500mg a day of choline.)

You can also find 'brain food' supplements providing a combination of different kinds of phospholipids, not just choline, but it's hard to get enough choline from these if your only other food sources are plant-based foods.

Your quick guide to essential fats and choline

We need both omega-6 and omega-3 fats, as well as phospholipids and choline.

- Too many omega-6 fats promote a deficiency of omega-3 fats, so limit sunflower and sesame seeds. Avoid them if you use tahini.
- Have a small handful daily of walnuts, pecan nuts, flax seeds, chia seeds, hemp seeds and/or a tablespoon of their oil or butter – they are all rich in omega-3.
- Eat one or two servings a day of dark green, leafy veg – especially those that grow in colder climates, such as kale, broccoli, Brussels sprouts, or a serving of seaweed as sources of both choline and omega-3.
- When using oils in cold food, such as salad dressings, use flax, rapeseed, walnut or hemp seed oil. Chia oil is also delicious, but it is not widely available.
- When using oils for cooking, use virgin rapeseed oil (not sunflower oil), or a fat such as coconut oil, or olive oil, which is almost saturated (mono-unsaturated).
- Have a serving, or two, of quinoa, beans or tofu every day, for choline.
- Supplement 250–300mg of DHA every day. Have a dessertspoon of high-PC lecithin, or two capsules of high-PC lecithin granules every day. These guidelines are especially important if you are planning a pregnancy, you are pregnant or breast-feeding.
- See Resources for a list of supplement suggestions.

Chapter 7

Control Your Sugar and Energy

Carbohydrates, our source of energy, come from plants. Plants literally make carbohydrates, which break down into glucose, which is the form of sugar our bodies run on. Although that is our primary fuel, we can also burn fats.

Plants absorb the energy from sunlight through their leaves and both use and effectively 'trap' this energy when they combine carbon and oxygen absorbed from the air (carbon dioxide, CO_2) with hydrogen and oxygen (H_2O) – water – taken in by their roots. This process makes carbohydrate. The by-product of this process is oxygen, which is expelled into the air. We eat and digest the carbohydrate, while breathing in the oxygen, and this helps to burn the carbohydrate and release what is in effect the sun's energy that was originally trapped in the making of the plant. How clever is that?

This is why everyone is dependent on the energy from plant foods, even if that energy has been stored in the animals that ate the plants. If there were no plants, there would be no humans. It's as simple as that.

Knowing this, there's good logic in going straight to the source for our energy. The simplest carbohydrate is glucose, which we call sugar, but there are actually lots of sugars. Fructose, the main sugar in fruit, can be converted into glucose in the liver. Sucrose (as in white sugar) is a molecule of glucose attached to a molecule of fructose. Maltose (as found in malted bread) is two glucose molecules combined that rapidly break down into glucose, which is also called dextrose. All of these are simple sugars, found in plants, that give you energy.

These sugars, however, release that potential energy into your bloodstream at different speeds, hence are described as either fast-releasing or slow-releasing. This is mainly dependent on how long it takes to turn them into glucose, which then enters the blood, which transports it to cells. This is important to know, because keeping your blood sugar steady is essential for good health. If we understand which foods are fast-releasing and which are slow-releasing, it gives us a benchmark to use to decide which carbohydrates are the best for us to eat on a regular basis for good health and to maintain a stable weight – and even for losing weight. The rate at which these carbohydrates raise blood glucose levels can be measured using the glycemic index, or GI, with glucose by definition scoring 100.

The glycemic index (GI) of sugars:	
Glucose, dextrose	100
Maltose	100 (glucose + glucose)
Rice syrup	98 (maltose)
Sucrose	65 (glucose + fructose)
Honey	58
Coconut sugar	54
Dates/date sugar	50

Grape juice nectar	50
Apple juice concentrate	44
Agave	19
Fructose	19
Xylose/xylitol	7

As you can see from the list above, these most basic sugars vary in the speed at which their glucose is released. The slower releasing the sugar, the more even your blood sugar level will remain. At the bottom of the list you can see the naturally occurring sugar, xylose, which is the slowest-releasing sugar. It is found in berries, cherries and plums. Further up the list is fructose, which is the main sugar contained in other fruits. Agave cactus nectar is also mainly fructose. Grain sugars, such as rice sugar (shown as rice syrup on the list), rapidly convert to glucose.

When looking at a healthy choice of added sugar, xylitol, the crystalline version of xylose, is probably the best. Nine teaspoons of xylitol has the same effect on your blood sugar as one teaspoon of sugar; however, in large quantities it can give you loose bowels. (Note that it is toxic to dogs, as is chocolate.)

The right kind of energy

If you're feeling tired, why not simply eat sugar? It contains plenty of energy, so when you eat it you will feel that energy kick. As I write this, I'm eating a piece of rye vollkornbrot – a German style of heavy bread containing whole grains –spread with sugar-free berry jam and some almond butter. But why not eat white bread and sugar-laden marmalade, which would provide much more instant sugar for energy?

There are two problems with doing this, and they illustrate exactly why you have to be careful on a plant-based diet to not go overboard on carbohydrates, choosing the ones you eat carefully and combining them with the right foods.

That slice of white bread and marmalade is like putting rocket fuel in a Mini and providing no engine oil. Firstly, a piece of refined bread, with the fibre removed, plus marmalade is about six teaspoons worth of sugar. In your bloodstream right now you have about three teaspoons of glucose. That's the amount you need at any point in time. Six teaspoons is more than you need, so when your body has extracted what your cells need for energy, the rest is dumped into storage as fat. Sugar makes you fat, especially around your middle. If you have excess fat around your belly you're eating too many carbs.

The second problem is that the efficient release of energy from carbs needs a whole family of nutrients, including B vitamins, vitamin C and the minerals magnesium, chromium, zinc, copper and iron. These are plentiful in the whole grain but not in refined white flour. That energy engine of yours will soon start sputtering as it runs out of vitamins, like an engine low on oil, which you'll experience as dips in mental and physical energy because you are not getting enough of the co-factor nutrients that drive the enzymes that turn the sugar into energy.

My rye bread, plus sugar-free berry jam and almond butter, is very different. Firstly, because I can see the whole grains in the bread I know that (a) all the nutrients in the grain are still in there; and (b) my teeth, through the action of chewing, and my digestive system are going to have to break down the whole grains and that will take time, thus releasing the natural sugars much more slowly. Furthermore, the fibre in the whole grains helps to nourish my microbiome and prevent constipation. Instead of getting a short burst of energy, I will feel energised and full for longer.

Then there's the jam. The sugar xylose, as we have seen, is found in berries, cherries and plums. It is very slow-releasing. Compared to pure glucose it raises blood sugar levels a ninth as much. And my sugar-free jam is basically just a compote of berries. Oranges, in marmalade, for example, are mainly fructose, so that's much faster releasing, plus marmalade, in common with all traditional preserves, contains a lot of sugar.

Now let's look at the almond butter. Almonds are rich in protein, and protein takes several hours to digest in the stomach. The carbs in the bread and the berry jam are digested, and their energy extracted, mainly further down your digestive system, in the small intestine, not the stomach. This delays the release of the sugars, giving me more sustained energy and making me feel fuller for longer. The presence of high-protein almonds, or peanuts, in a sugar-free nut butter will further slow the release of the sugars in the bread and the jam. Again, that's going to keep me energised for much longer and, without that sudden spike in blood sugar, there's no big excess of glucose to dump into storage as fat. This way I stay lean and keep my energy level stable.

If I eat too many carbs, especially fast-releasing carbs on their own, without protein, I'm going to have blood sugar highs and lows, and the lows will trigger hunger, so I'll keep craving more carbs. If you keep feeling hungry, and craving carbs, you're eating too many carbs, or the wrong kind, in the wrong combinations.

Why GL is the best measure

There's a simple tool that you can use to optimise your energy and your nutrient intake, without getting fat, while following a plant-based diet. It's called GL, short for 'glycemic *load*'. A food that is low-GL will keep your blood sugar level even, whereas a high-GL food will cause high spikes, followed by rebound blood sugar and energy dips, triggering hunger. If a food, for example my whole-rye bread, contains fibre, this lowers the GL. And if the food contains protein, such as beans, that will also lower its GL.

Whereas the *GI* of a food (as illustrated in the sugars list earlier) simply *defines* the kind of sugar contained within it – whether fast- or slow-releasing – the *GL* of a food factors in *how much* actual available sugar is in the food *portion* that you ate and how fast-releasing it is. The GL represents the *quality*: the GI multiplied by the *quantity* of available carbs.

Example: the GI of white bread is 70. The GI of 50 slices of white bread is also 70. A slice of bread has 14g of available carbs; so the GL of a slice of white bread is .70 × 14 = 10GLs. The GL of two slices of bread is therefore 20GLs.

Once you know the GL of a serving of any food, a meal or a recipe, you will know what it's going to do to your blood sugar. The GL also predicts how much insulin (the fat-storing hormone) is going to be released.[22] I've calculated the GLs of all the recipes in Part 3. Later in this chapter you'll find the GLs for accompaniments such as vegetables, pasta, rice and breads.

How many GLs should you aim for?

As a guideline, if you eat 60GLs a day, you'll stay the same weight. If you eat 45GLs, you'll lose weight. If you eat 80GLs or more, you'll gain weight. That's assuming an average amount of exercise. Now, of course, if you're running a half marathon a day, you'll need more – at least 80GLs.

Did our ancestors eat a high-carb diet?

One of the big debates today in diet and nutrition circles is whether it is better to eat a very low-carb diet (for example 20 per cent or less of calories), as advocated by high-fat 'keto' meat eaters, or a rather high-carb diet (for example 70 per cent or more of calories), an extreme version of which would be the diet followed by fruitarians. I advocate something in the middle (50–55 per cent of calories from slow-releasing carbs, 15–20 per cent from protein and around 30 per cent from fat) for reasons that will become clear.

Advocates of high-carb diets cite the long living Tsimané tribe in the Peruvian Amazon, who are among the very few who still follow a more prehistoric lifestyle. As we saw on page 26 in Chapter 2, they obtain 72 per cent of their calories from unrefined, high-fibre (and hence low-GL) carbohydrates, and protein comprises 14 per cent of their diet, mainly from lean animal meat and fish. Their fat intake is low – just 14 per cent – far lower than the average Western diet. They have the lowest risk of heart disease in the world: even those over the age of 75 have virtually no cardiovascular problems or hardening of the arteries. The Hadza in Tanzania have a very similar diet, and they are just as healthy. However, before you decide to follow suit with your carbohydrate intake, bear in mind that both of these tribes burn a lot of calories through exercise. The average Tsimané man hunts for around six to seven hours each day, while the average woman gathers and prepares food for four to five hours. All this is hard physical activity, so they need more carbs for energy.

Also, their carbs are from whole foods, full of fibre, hence low GL. The trouble with many vegan packaged foods, on the other hand, although they might sound good, is that they use natural sweeteners such as dates, raisins and bananas, or cool-sounding sugars such as coconut sugar, all of which are high GL. It's just as easy to gain weight on a vegan diet as a non-vegan diet if you eat too many carbs, and that's very easy to do, as the following box illustrates.

Reading the label

Let's take a look at two snack bars as an illustration of why it's easy to eat too many carbs while aiming for a healthy vegan diet. The critical bit to read on any food label is the total grams of carbohydrates, what quantity is sugar, and the fibre content. Have a look at the nutritional info for the two snack bars below, with these measures in bold.

A Nākd Cocoa Crunch bar has 14.2g of carbs, 12.9g of which are sugar. A teaspoon of sugar is 4g, so we're looking at more than three teaspoons of sugar. (Government guidelines recommend no more than five in a day.)

Nutritional info

Typical values	Per 100g	Per 30g
Energy	1469kJ	440kJ
	351kcal	105kcal
Fat	8.8g	2.6g
of which saturates	2.0g	0.6g
Carbohydrate	47.2g	14.2g
of which sugars	42.9g	12.9g
Fibre	6.3g	1.9g
Protein	18.4g	5.5g
Salt	0.6g	0.2g

The next thing to look at is the ingredients list. Foods have to be listed in order of the largest quantity, down to the smallest quantity. The ingredients for the Nākd Cocoa Crunch are: 'Dates (43%), Soya Protein Crunchies (soya, tapioca starch, salt) (16%), Raisins

(16%), Cashews (15%), Cocoa (5%), Apple Juice Concentrate (4%) and a hint of natural flavouring.' Dates and raisins, making 59 per cent of the bar, are all pretty fast-releasing sugars. To their credit they've put in the soya protein crunch and nuts. Remember, protein and fibre slow down the release of carbs, hence lowering the GL. Each bar has 1.9g of fibre and 5.5g of protein. This is quite typical of many of the bars that state they are 'natural' or have 'no added sugar'.

Let's compare this to Pulsin's Plant-Based Keto Chocolate Fudge and Peanut Bar (see Resources).

Nutritional info

	Per Serving (50g)	Per 100g
Energy	1033kJ	2066kJ
	247kcal	494kcal
Fat	16.0g	32.0g
of which saturated	5.9g	11.8g
Carbohydrate	8.6g	17.1g
of which sugars	1.9g	3.8g
of which polyols	4.5g	9.0g
Fibre	9.3g	18.6g
Protein	12.6g	25.2g
Salt	0.28g	0.57g

It contains 8.6g of carbs of which 1.9g are sugar – that's less than half a teaspoon of sugar. It's got 9.3g of fibre, more than six times the other bar, and double the protein at 12.6g, which will further slow down the release of the sugars. Its sweet taste is due to the use of xylitol, the crystalline version of the sugar in berries, and chicory root fibre, a natural source of inulin, which tastes sweet but has no effect on blood sugar level, hence 0GL. It uses peanuts and pea protein to increase the protein level.

The simplest way to sum all this up is the GL score. Pulsin's 50g bar I estimate to be around 1GL, whereas the Nākd 30g bar is going to be close to 9GLs, despite being much smaller. The Nākd bar is no worse than most vegan bars. It just shows how foods that appear to be low in sugar can be loaded with fast-releasing, high-GL carbs.

Beware disguised sugars

There are many fast-releasing sugars dressed up to appear good for you, from date sugar to coconut sugar (which is sometimes called coconut blossom sugar). Apple juice concentrate is slightly better for you than grape juice concentrate, but of all the liquid sweeteners, agave, from the agave cactus, is the best. Xylitol, called a sugar alcohol, is the best crystalline sugar, as we have seen. There are other less natural sugar alcohols (all ending in '-ol'), such as erythritol. Inulin, derived from chicory root fibre, is not a sugar but a fibre, and feeds the bacteria in your gut. It's the best sweetener, with no GL, but some people experience bloating if they eat too much of it. Agave is a liquid, so it is sometimes useful to drizzle over foods, but please use this in very small amounts nevertheless.

The basic low-GL principles

To benefit from eating the low-GL way, apply the following basic principles:

1. Eat 60GLs a day, or 45GLs to lose weight.
2. Combine protein foods with carbohydrate foods.
3. Eat little and often – three 10GL meals (for weight loss) or 15GL meals (for maintenance), two 5GL snacks, plus 5GLs for a drink or dessert.

Neither fat nor protein substantially affects blood sugar, but, as you've now discovered, carbs do, so you need to prioritise eating slow carbs in the right quantities, to optimise your health, weight and energy. The glucose level in your blood determines your hunger more than anything else, and it's hunger that drives overeating and weight gain.

In visual terms, half your plate should comprise of vegetables and/or low-GL fruit; one-quarter protein-rich foods; and one-quarter carbohydrate-rich foods (see the illustration overleaf). If you prefer to think in terms of calories, this equates to around 15–20 per cent of your total calorific intake from protein, 30 per cent from fat and 50–55 per cent from carbohydrates – but you won't be counting calories.

Plate showing proportions of foods for weight maintenance

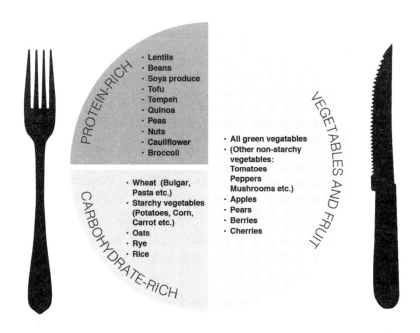

I'm giving you the guidelines for weight maintenance, but if you want to lose weight, your meal plate will look more like the dotted lines in the plate on the facing page, with fewer carbohydrate-rich and more protein-rich foods. This is because most plant-based sources of protein also contain a significant amount of carbs. This isn't a bad thing – it just means that you're getting two key macronutrients from one food.

Plate showing reduced carbs for weight loss

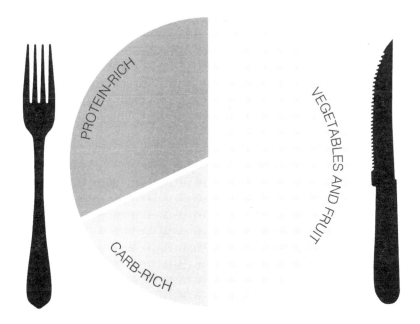

In the above version, although it looks as if your carb intake is less than a quarter of the plate, the food you eat for protein, such as beans, lentils or quinoa, also contains carbs so, in reality, you'll be getting *more* carbs than what's on a quarter of your plate. Also, the vegetables contain carbs, albeit very low-GL carbs. The only vegan protein-rich foods that don't provide so much in the way of carbs are soya produce, chickpeas (or hummus), lentils, Quorn, nuts and seeds. These are foods with a protein-to-carb ratio of 0.6 or above in the chart overleaf. A ratio of 1 means that there's the same amount of protein as carbs in the food; for example, soya mince has twice as much protein as carbs with a protein–carb ratio of 2 whereas brown rice has ten times more carbs than protein with a protein–carb ratio of 0.1.

Plant-based protein foods and their protein–carb ratios

In Chapter 5, on page 72, you saw how much of a protein-rich food you would need to eat to achieve 15g of protein. This is what you're aiming for three times a day. Now, in the chart below, you'll see the same foods but this time with the percentage of calories from protein and the percentage of calories from carbs, going from the highest protein–carb ratio to the lowest. I've also added rice and other grains, since these do provide protein, and also as a comparison.

Protein, carbs and protein–carb ratio

Food	% Protein	% Carb	Protein–carb ratio
Tofu	41%	9%	4.6
Hummus	35%	17%	2.1
Soya mince	58%	28%	2
Tempeh	32%	19%	1.7
Quorn	44%	36%	1.2
Peanuts	14%	15%	0.9
Nuts (almonds, raw)	13%	15%	0.9
Pumpkin seeds	13%	16%	0.8
Almond milk	10%	15%	0.7
Soya milk	26%	42%	0.6
Chia seeds	18%	35%	0.5
Lentils	27%	70%	0.4

Food	% Protein	% Carb	Protein–carb ratio
Kidney beans	24%	73%	0.3
Black-eyed beans	23%	74%	0.3
Baked beans	22%	77%	0.3
Quinoa	15%	70%	0.2
Wheat/barley/ rye/oats	13–15%	70–82%	0.2
Rice, brown long grain	8%	85%	0.1
Oat milk	8%	57%	0.1

In the table above you can see that the higher the percentage in the first column, the more protein that food will give you. The lower the percentage in the second column, the fewer carbs that food will give you. In the third column, anything above 1 means that the food has more protein than carbs.

What this means for you is that you will be reducing carbs and also achieving your protein needs if you do the following, for example:

- Eat more nuts or seeds and less oat flakes, using soya or carb-free almond milk instead of oat milk in your breakfast.
- Eat more beans or lentils and less rice in a main meal.
- Eat tofu, tempeh or Quorn for your main meal protein with lots of veg.
- Eat more nuts and seeds and less fruit for a snack, or perhaps have hummus with raw veg or a couple of oatcakes.

Don't worry about fats – it's the GL that counts

The remaining percentage points in the table above, out of 100 per cent, come from fat. Looking at nuts and seeds as an example, pumpkin seeds have 13 per cent of calories from protein, 16 per cent from carbs and therefore 71 per cent from fat. They are high in fat, whereas black-eyed beans, which are 23 per cent protein, 74 per cent carbs and therefore 3 per cent fat, are very low. (Some foods, such as peanuts, are not naturally high in fat but are cooked in oil, hence their high fat content.) Our focus is not on fats in this chapter, but on learning how to balance sugars in your diet, which drives your appetite. There is also no need to avoid the healthy fats in nuts and seeds. Fats are not 'bad' for you. It wouldn't matter if you increased your fat intake, as long as you reduced your carb intake accordingly. Of course, ideally, choose carefully and eat foods that provide the essential fats discussed in Chapter 6.

The key factor to remember is to control the glycemic load (GL) of the carbs you eat – 10–15GLs for a main meal (for weight loss or maintenance) and 5GLs for snacks, drinks and desserts. Remember, it's the GL that determines your blood sugar balance, and consequently insulin release, and too much insulin and fluctuating blood sugar levels are behind almost every major disease, from obesity to diabetes and heart disease. Let's see how this works, starting with the half-plate vegetable portion for a main meal.

Vegetables

Half a plate of non-starchy veg (such as greens, peppers, tomatoes and other common salad ingredients), representing roughly two servings, is about 3GLs. Most vegetables are between 1 and 2GLs per serving, with salad vegetables being 1GL. Vegetables are the main part of your plant-based diet. They are rich in vitamins, minerals, antioxidants and polyphenols. Broccoli and cauliflower are also quite rich in protein, so they are a good food to include in your diet. Vegetables are also carbs, so given your daily 10–15GL allowance, less the 3GLs from vegetables, you can have a 7–12GL portion for the carbohydrate-rich quarter of your plate, for example wholewheat spaghetti, brown rice or potatoes – or beans or quinoa if you are using them as carbs, rather than your protein food (see below). I'll show you how much makes up a 7 or 12GL portion of these kinds of carb-rich foods on pages 115–16.

Some veg contain higher carbs, and these are also listed in the carb section of the meal plate on page 108. These include potatoes, sweet potatoes, sweetcorn, carrots, beetroot, parsnips and broad beans. If you eat a portion of them, as you would potatoes, they count as a carbohydrate-rich food in that quarter of your plate. If you add a little to your veg portion, perhaps grating some beetroot or carrot on your salad, you won't be getting much more in the way of GLs or carbs, so don't worry about that. If you ate a medium-sized carrot (5GLs) with some hummus for a snack that's OK, too.

High-GL vegetables

Food	Serving size in grams	Looks like	GLs
Carrots	80	1 small	3
Green peas	80	1½ tbsp	3
Pumpkin/squash	80	2 tbsp	3
Beetroot	80	2 small	5
Swede	150	⅓ swede	7

Food	Serving size in grams	Looks like	GLs
Sweet potato wedges	50	1 small serving	8
Banana/plantain, green	120	1 very small	8
Broad beans	80	2 tbsp	9
Sweet potato and carrot mash	50	1 serving	10
Parsnips	80	1 medium	12
Sweetcorn, on the cob, boiled	150	⅓ cob	14
Yam	150	1 medium	13
Boiled potato	150	3 small	14
Microwaved potato	150	3 small	14

If, for example, you'd like to lose some weight, go easy on sweet potatoes, sweetcorn, potatoes, parsnips, broad beans, carrots and beetroot. The 'sweet' in the name is an obvious giveaway in some of these veg.

Getting your carb portion right

How much of the carb-rich foods in a main meal do you need to eat to achieve the goal of 7GLs (for weight loss) or 12GLs (for maintenance) of carbs? This is really about knowledge, as you can have twice as much wholewheat bulgur wheat as you can wholewheat pasta or brown rice.

Portions of carb-rich foods

Food	7GLs serving size	12GLs serving size
Kamut wholewheat bulgur	Large serving (190g/6¾oz)	Very large serving (325g/11½oz)
Pumpkin/squash	Large serving (185g/6½oz)	Very large serving (316g/11oz)
Carrot	1 large (160g/5¾oz)	2 medium (273g/10oz)
Swede	Large serving (150g/5½oz)	Very large serving (256g/9oz)
Quinoa	Large serving (130g/4¾oz)	Very large serving (222g/8oz)
Beetroot	Large serving (110g/3¾oz)	2 beetroots (188g/6½oz)
Cornmeal	Medium serving (115g/4oz)	Large serving (197g/7oz)
Pearl barley	Small serving (95g/3¼oz)	1 serving (162g/5¾oz)
Wholewheat pasta	½ serving (85g/3oz) cooked weight	1 serving (145g/5oz)
White pasta	⅓ serving (65g/2¼oz) cooked weight	Small serving (111g/3¾oz)
Buckwheat noodles	⅓ serving (50g/1¾oz)	½ serving (86g/3oz)
Buckwheat	Small serving (70g/2½oz) cooked weight	1 serving (120g/4¼oz)

Food	7GLs serving size	12GLs serving size
Brown rice	Small serving (70g/2½oz) cooked weight	1 serving (120g/4¼oz)
White rice	⅓ serving (45g/1½oz) cooked weight	Very small serving (75g/2¾oz)
Boiled potato	3 small (75g/2¾oz)	3 medium (128g/4½oz)
Baked potato	½ (60g/2⅛oz)	1 medium (100g/3½oz)
French fries	Tiny portion (45g/2½oz)	Small portion (75g/2¾oz)
Sweet potato	½ (60g/2⅛oz)	Small potato (100g/3½oz)
Couscous	⅓ serving (45g/1½oz), soaked weight	½ serving (75g/2¾oz)
Broad beans	Small serving (30g/1oz)	1 serving (50g/1¾oz)
Corn on the cob	½ cob (60g/2⅛oz)	a small cob (100g/3½oz)
Millet	½ cup, cooked (60g/2⅛oz)	1 cup (100g/3½oz)

As you can see, there are some high and some low 'value' foods in this list. The stated portions of kamut khorosan bulgur (an ancient wheat that takes only eight minutes to cook) and quinoa (which takes 15 minutes) will certainly fill you up. The former is delicious on its own, whereas the latter ideally needs some sort of flavouring, but it is a very good source of protein. Wholewheat pasta and brown rice are both much better options than the white alternatives, but the portion size is still much smaller than bulgur or quinoa. Similarly, swedes, carrots and squashes are all preferable to potatoes. And boiled potato is better than baked potato, which is better than French fries.

As we saw above, some plant-based protein-rich foods also contain a lot of carbs. Beans and lentils are a case in point. Therefore, foods such as beans can meet both your protein and carb portion requirements. An example would be a vegan chilli using black-eyed beans or the more traditional kidney beans, served with half a plate of veg. If you look at the chart below, half a can of black-eyed beans per person would not only provide 12GLs but also enough protein. If you used the more traditional kidney beans two-thirds of a can per person would give enough protein on its own, plus 7GLs.

In the table below you can see what quantity of various beans you would need to eat to achieve 15g of protein – the ideal amount for a meal. It also shows the amount that provides 7GLs (for weight loss) or 12GLs (for maintenance). Obviously I'm not suggesting you eat numerous cans of beans – it simply demonstrates the degree to which the carb content of beans varies.

Food serving sizes for 15g of protein

Food	Serving sizes	
15g protein	7GLs	12GLs
Soya beans ⅕ can (40g)	4 cans (1.05kg)	7 cans (1.78kg)
Peas ¼ can (65g)	2 cans (525g)	3 cans (892g)
Pinto beans ¼ can (65g)	1 can (262g)	1¾ cans (445g)

Food	Serving sizes	
15g protein	**7GLs**	**12GLs**
Borlotti beans ¼ can (65g)	1 can (262g)	1¾ cans (445g)
Lentils ⅔ can (170g)	<1 can (210g)	1½ cans (357g)
Butter beans ⅔ can (190g)	<1 can (175g)	1¼ cans (297g)
Split peas ¼ can (60g)	<1 can (175g)	1¼ cans (297g)
Baked beans 1⅓ cans (310g)	⅔ can (150g)	1 can (255g)
Kidney beans ⅔ can (175g)	⅔ can (150g)	1 can (255g)
Chickpeas ¾ can (164g)	½ can (132g)	1 can (224g)
Flageolet beans ¾ can (210g)	½ can (116g)	⅔ can (197g)
Haricot beans 1 can (250g)	⅓ can (87g)	½ can (148g)
Black-eyed beans ½ can (165g)	⅓ can (87g)	½ can (148g)

The serving size of cans is approximate. A 400g can provides about 240g of beans.

The recipes in Part 3 are all calculated to be in the right GL ballpark for either weight loss (7GLs + veg) or maintenance (12GLs + veg). It's good to understand how it all works so that you can work out your own recipes and menus, but a simple alternative is to get used to making the recipes in the book then, instinctively, you'll get an idea of the appropriate serving sizes when you start making meal variations.

Of course, in reality, we tend to serve what we think will fill us up. If you are full, stop eating! You'll find the GL-friendly vegan recipes in Part 3 are very filling, as well as nourishing.

Breakfasts

Now that you understand the principles for a main meal we can apply these easily to your breakfast. For breakfast, as for all meals, aim for 10GLs (for weight loss) or 15GLs (for maintenance). If you choose to eat a cereal for breakfast, let's assume you have it with a 5GL portion of fruit, leaving 5GLs or 10GLs (weight loss or maintenance) for the cereal. Here's what a 5GL or 10GL cereal portion looks like. As you can see, the best 'value' cereal in terms of satisfying your hunger, are oat flakes, either cooked (as in porridge) or eaten raw (like cornflakes). Basically, you can eat as much as you like, given that two cups will fill anybody up.

GLs for breakfast cereals

Cereal	5GLs serving size	10GLs serving size
Oat flakes	1 cup/95g/3¼oz	1 bowl or 2 cups/190g/6¾oz
All-Bran	1 serving (½ bowl or 1 cup/60g/2⅛oz)	1 bowl or 2 cups/120g/4¼oz
Unsweetened muesli	1 small serving (less than ½ bowl or ¾ cup/75g/2¾oz	A small bowl or 1 cup/150g/5½oz
Alpen	½ serving (¼ bowl or ½ cup/50g/1¾oz)	½ bowl or 1 cup/100g/3½oz
Raisin Bran	½ serving (¼ bowl or ½ cup/30g/1oz)	½ bowl or 1 cup/60g/2⅛oz

Cereal	5GLs serving size	10GLs serving size
Weetabix	1 biscuit	2 biscuits
Lizi's Original Low-GL Granola	½ bowl or 1 cup/55g/2oz	1 bowl or 2 cups/110g/3¾oz

Now add some fruit as a natural sweetener. As you can see below, berries are the best choice, or you can have chopped pear, apple or peach.

GLs for fruits

	5GLs
Berries	1 large punnet
Plums	4
Cherries	1 small punnet
Pear	1
Grapefruit	1
Orange	1
Apple	1 small (fits in the palm of your hand)
Peach	1 small
Banana	Less than half
Melon/watermelon	1 slice
Raisins	10
Dates	1

Applying the principle of always eating protein with carbs, now add some nuts or seeds. This could be a small handful of chia, flax, pumpkin seeds or almonds, walnuts or pecan nuts, or perhaps a mixture of both. Also, you want to pick a higher protein milk, such as soya or almond, providing they're unsweetened. Oat milk contains more carbs than protein.

There are lots of GL-balanced breakfasts in Part 3, including Wild Mushrooms on Toast, Porridge with Almonds and Goji Berries, Chia Pancakes with Pear Compote, Apple and Hazelnut Granola, Bircher Muesli and low-GL Banana Muffins. Each combine a source of protein, such as chia, with a low-GL carb food, such as oats in the pancake recipe.

You can also make low-GL smoothies applying the same principles. When you make a smoothie, use the whole fruit, not just the juice, and perhaps add some greens to keep the GL down. Increase the protein by adding a nut butter and/or pea protein and ground seeds. Be careful not to use too much fruit juice, if any (see page 125). Here's an example of ingredients you can use to experiment with and make a variety of smoothies according to your taste preferences. A smoothie such as this is a good breakfast option.

- Pea protein (see Resources) and/or 1 tablespoon of almond or peanut butter (sugar-free)
- Ground nuts (such as almonds) or seeds (such as chia)
- Frozen or fresh berries with an optional ½ banana (which can be chopped and frozen beforehand to make a cold smoothie)
- A handful of baby spinach, wheatgrass, barley grass or spirulina
- A cup (250ml/9fl oz) of nut milk (almond or soya is the lowest GL)
- Water or coconut water
- Cinnamon

Another good snack or breakfast is my low-GL Get Up & Go with Carboslow shake. The combination of a 30g serving with a nut milk and a handful of berries is 8GLs, or 10GLs with oat milk, and is ideal for breakfast. Get Up & Go achieves this low GL by using chicory root fibre and xylitol as the sweeteners. It also contains a super-soluble fibre called glucomannan, which helps to lower the GL. With a handful of berries and a carb-free milk it totals 5GLs, so that's good for a snack as well as a breakfast.

Snacks

As explained earlier, the aim of eating low-GL is to achieve an even blood sugar level by eating little and often. In this way your blood sugar level, insulin and appetite stay on an even keel. Although some people prefer to have fewer meals, such as two meals a day and no snacks, most studies show that this doesn't work as well for most people. They end up eating more. It's an individual thing, but most research does confirm that grazing (having breakfast, and two meals, plus healthy snacks) is healthier for you than gorging (having one or two big meals in the day).[23] Vegans eating in this way, also with some regular fasting, tend to be the healthiest, with stable weight.[24]

Aside from your main meals you have a daily allowance of 5GLs × 3, designed to deliver a mid-morning snack, a mid-afternoon snack and 5GLs for drinks or desserts. The mid-afternoon snack is particularly important because, if you come home at the end of the day with a low blood sugar you'll unconsciously gravitate towards fast-sugar foods. Resistance is weaker later in the day. By having a low-GL afternoon snack you'll make better choices in the evening. The ideal snack is one that provides no more than 5GLs and also some protein. Remember: eating protein with carbs slows down the release of sugars from the carbs.

The simplest snack food is fruit. On the previous page you saw what a 5GL portion of fruit is. Berries, plums and cherries, being high in xylose, are your best-value fruit snacks as far as GLs are concerned. Berries include strawberries, raspberries, blueberries, blackberries and any others that you can get your hands on in season, or buy them frozen. You can further slow down the score of these fruits by eating them with a few almonds or walnuts or a small handful of pumpkin seeds. Almonds are one of the best nuts, because they have the most protein compared with calories. Pumpkin seeds are also high in protein and have some omega-3 fats. Hemp seeds do, too, but they are too hard to crunch. Walnuts are best for omega-3, followed by pecan nuts. Flax seeds and chia seeds are good but not so easy to eat. You could, however, use them in whole fruit smoothies. Frozen berries and sliced and frozen banana defrost in the blender when used for smoothies and make a nice cooling drink.

Another snack option would be some kind of bread with a protein-based spread such as hummus or a nut butter – almond or peanut for example – but make sure they're sugar-free. Hummus is also good with raw veg, such as celery or carrot.

A slice of any of the bread servings below with either hummus or another bean pâté or a nut butter gives you the right kind of low carbohydrate with some protein to keep your blood sugar level even.

Oatcakes, and oats in general, are excellent as far as weight and blood sugar are concerned. Oats contain beta-glucan, a type of fibre that helps to slow down the release of glucose into the blood, lessen insulin response and also lower cholesterol and heart disease risk. Of all the grains, it's the best for losing weight, and for controlling your blood sugar.[25]

Watch out when buying oatcakes, though, as many contain sugar. Sugar-free, organic rough oatcakes are preferable. Some also use palm fruit oil (which contains unsaturated fat) from sustainable farms, as opposed to palm oil (which is higher in saturated fat). I like Nairn's as they meet these criteria and are widely available.

Bread and oatcakes

	5GLs
Rough oatcakes	2½ biscuits
Fine oatcakes	2 biscuits
Pumpernickel-style rye bread	1 thin slice
Sourdough rye bread	1 thin slice
Rye wholemeal bread (yeasted)	½ slice
Wheat wholemeal bread (yeasted)	½ slice
White, high fibre bread (yeasted)	less than ½ slice
Croissant, or bagel	less than ½

Here is a selection of five low-GL snacks to choose from:

- A piece of fruit, plus 5 almonds or 2 teaspoons of pumpkin seeds.
- A thin slice of rye bread or 2 oatcakes and half a small tub of hummus (150g/5½oz).
- A thin slice of rye bread or 2 oatcakes and sugar-free nut butter.
- Crudités (a raw carrot, pepper, cucumber or celery) and hummus or any bean pâté.
- Crudités and vegan cream cheese.
- A small sugar-free coconut or soya yoghurt (150g/5½oz), plus berries.
- A low-GL bar (See Reading the label, page 104, and Resources, page 261).

There are a number of snack recipes in Part 3 starting on page 171, including Pine Nut and Sun-Dried Pepper Hummus, Red Pepper and Cucumber Salsa, Guacamole, Sun-Dried Tomato and Black Olive Pesto, Aubergine Pâté and Pumpkin Seed Pesto.

Cold drinks and juices

A good rule of thumb is to *eat* fruit, not to *drink* it. The main sugar in fruit is fructose. Once you consume above six teaspoons (for women) or nine teaspoons (for men) fructose turns into harmful fats (triglycerides) in the blood and suppresses your appetite control. Many processed and canned drinks exceed this amount.

Nature only ever makes fructose – fruit sugar – with fibre. The fibre slows down the release of sugar, so eat the whole fruit or make a smoothie using the whole fruit, *not* a juice where the fibre is removed.

Generally I avoid fruit juice. My only exception to this is Blueberry Active (made from pure blueberries) or Cherry Active (made from Montmorency cherries), both of which are relatively low GL and very high in antioxidants (see Resources). All commercial fruit juices, whether concentrated or freshly squeezed, have a relatively high GL because the fibre has been removed. The best is probably cloudy apple juice, although even this should be drunk diluted – half juice:half water or, even better, two-thirds water to one-third juice.

The following table indicates 5GL portions for a variety of drinks. Remember: aim to stick to the 5GL allowance for drinks or desserts. If you spend it on drinks, go easy on desserts.

Drinks

	5GLs
Tomato juice	500ml (18fl oz)
Carrot juice	Small glass
Grapefruit juice, unsweetened	Small glass
Apple juice, unsweetened	Small glass, diluted 50:50 with water
Orange juice, unsweetened	Small glass, diluted 50:50 with water, or freshly squeezed juice of 1 orange
Blueberry Active	20ml (approx.1 tbsp) of concentrate
Cherry Active	20ml (approx.1 tbsp) of concentrate
Pineapple juice	½ small glass, diluted 50:50 with water
Cranberry juice	½ small glass, diluted 50:50 with water
Grape juice	2cm (1in) in a glass – avoid!

Stay away from all fizzy and sweetened drinks as well as sugar-sweetened cordials.

A good rule of thumb is to have no more than one glass of juice each day, diluting it as need be, so that you never have more than 5GLs in the course of the day. You could have either a small glass of carrot juice, *or* the juice of one orange *or* a small glass of diluted apple juice. Always drink slowly – sip rather than gulp – as this helps to retard the release of the sugars in the juice (as does diluting). This is also a good rule of thumb for children, otherwise you are helping them develop a sweet tooth and rotting their teeth in the process. Xylose, in berries, protects their teeth. The best drink to get used to is water.

Hot drinks

There's no GL in tea, coffee or herb teas – well, a tiny bit in fruit teas – but there's a lot of hidden sugar in speciality coffees depending on what else is added. One recent example was of a Christmas drink from a well-known coffee chain: a large-sized (590ml) caramel hot chocolate with whipped cream and oat milk, which was found to contain the equivalent of 23 teaspoons of sugar! Other coffee chains had similar sugar-laden festive drinks. The point is that it's what you add to tea or coffee that bumps up the sugar content. In coffee shops many of the vegan milks have added sugar. Ask for one that doesn't. Coconut milk is usually the sweetest. Sugar-free soya or almond milk is usually the best. Oat milk, while there's no sugar added, has a higher GL than unsweetened soya milk. If you need to sweeten a drink, add a little xylitol, or raw cacao for a chocolate flavour, and cinnamon, which is good for blood sugar balance. One teaspoon of xylitol is less than 0.5GLs.

Low-GL desserts

If you eat a lot of desserts, or if you are insulin-resistant (which affects omnivores, vegetarians and vegans equally), you will probably crave something sweet at the end of each meal. It is very important to break this habit because, if you don't, it will keep your blood sugar level see sawing. It takes only three days in most cases to stop the craving, however. Also, it takes some time for your appetite to register satiety, so don't dive into a dessert after your main meal. Wait a while. Even better would be to have the lunchtime dessert, perhaps the plum crumble on page 256, for your afternoon snack, going for a walk in between.

You'll find wonderful recipes for low-GL desserts in Part 3, starting on page 246, including Chocolate Crunchies, Coconut and Pineapple Sorbet, Apricot and Ginger Flapjack Bites, Plum Crumble with Cinnamon and Oats, and Almond Shortbread.

Generally it's better not to have desserts when you are eating out unless your vegan restaurant is switched on to lower sugar options. Most vegan desserts are high in sugar. You can have a 5GL dessert with your meal and leave out one of your snacks, but having the snack is better, because this way you will be grazing rather than gorging. This helps to keep your blood sugar, energy and weight even.

Your quick guide to low-GL eating

Become GL savvy by avoiding fast-releasing added sugary ingredients, even 'natural' sugars from dates, grape juice and coconut sugar or nectar. If you need a sweetener, use xylitol or agave.

- Aim for 60GLs a day (45GLs for weight loss).
- Graze rather than gorge – with 15GLs for a main meal and 5GLs for snacks.
- Always eat protein foods with carbs.
- Go easy on high-GL veg such as potatoes and sweet potatoes, and bread, and high-GL fruit such as bananas, grapes and raisins.
- Eat fruit, don't drink it – whole fruit smoothies being the exception.

Chapter 8

Vitamin Essentials

Vitamins are essential compounds that we have to get from food. Without them nothing works: your skin becomes dry and scaly, your teeth loosen and your gums bleed (from scurvy due to a lack of vitamin C); your energy plummets (B vitamins make energy); your bones get weak (vitamin D makes healthy bones); and your immune system can't fight off infections (vitamins A, B, C and D are all needed for a healthy immune system).

The definition of a vitamin is that it's essential for your health. They are divided into water-soluble and fat-soluble vitamins: the water-soluble vitamins are all the B vitamins and vitamin C; the fat-soluble vitamins are vitamins A, D and E. All the water-soluble vitamins are available from plant foods, with the exception of vitamin B12, which is made by bacteria and is found only in animal products in any significant quantity (all animal products provide B12). It is therefore essential to supplement vitamin B12 on a vegan diet. Vitamin A, although richest in animal foods, can be derived from its precursor, beta-carotene, which is plentiful in plants such as carrots, butternut squash and greens. Vitamin E is rich in seafood but also in the oils of nuts, seeds and grains. Vitamin D, although richest in eggs and fish, is also made in the skin in the presence of sunlight; hence, adequate sun exposure is needed. Vitamin D is therefore hard to get enough of, especially in winter, without supplementation. Most vitamin D in supplements is derived from lanolin in wool, although it can be synthesised, hence vegan.

Why you need vitamin B12

Vitamin B12 makes protein, helps red blood cells to carry oxygen, is vital for energy, and is essential for making DNA, building nerves and the brain, and one of the most critical processes in the body, methylation, depends on it. Methylation controls genetic expression (explained in Chapter 1), makes the phospholipids discussed in Chapter 6, balances hormones and neurotransmitters, and affects how you think and feel – and much more besides. Being a 'good methylator', which means having an optimal supply of B vitamins, is a fundamental pillar of being healthy and disease-proofing your life. That's why poor methylation is linked to an increased risk of cancer, heart disease, autoimmune diseases, osteoporosis and mental illness. Without healthy methylation, blood levels of a toxic amino acid called homocysteine rise, which is associated with pregnancy problems, memory loss, poor mood, increased anxiety and ultimately nerve dysfunction, which is experienced as loss of sensation in the extremities (peripheral neuropathy). Every few seconds there are a billion methylation reactions in your body and brain, all dependent on B12. (See Further Reading for more on the topic of homocysteine.)

As mentioned, vitamin B12 is vital for gene expression, which is the term used to describe the way in which our genes are turned up or down, either to become more or less active. As we saw on page 15, about half of women who have the BRCA gene, which increases the risk of breast cancer, get breast cancer, but half don't. One reason for the difference could be connected to eating soya or dairy: soya dampens down the BRCA gene and is associated with reducing cancer cell growth whereas dairy products promote cancer cell growth. This might mean that vegans have a lower risk of breast cancer. But if you lack the methylating B vitamins, such as B12, your risk goes up even further, so if you are a vegan it's important to supplement B12, since this is one vitamin that you can't get from vegan foods alone.

Regardless of whether you're vegan, B12 insufficiency is quite common, especially during pregnancy and in young mothers, and in those over 60, affecting at least one in five. Studies world-wide find that between 11 and 90 per cent of vegetarians have B12 deficiency (there are no detailed studies about vegans at this time). In countries such as India, where lifelong vegetarians form a high proportion of the population, up to 71 per cent of pregnant women are B12 deficient.[1] A study in the US found low levels of B12 in the breast milk in 19 per cent of vegans, 18 per cent of vegetarians and 15 per cent of non-vegetarians. Those supplementing B12, however, had higher B12 levels in their breast milk.[2] In another US study of vegetarian adults the use of B12 supplements or the use of B12 fortified milk substitutes were good predictors of sufficient blood B12 levels.[3]

Vitamin B12 in food has to combine with a stomach secretion called 'intrinsic factor' to be absorbed. Some people don't make enough intrinsic factor and hence are prone to pernicious anaemia, which is one cause of B12 deficiency, and have to either supplement a lot more or have B12 injections. (See Resources for information about The Pernicious Anaemia Society if you suspect you might have an issue.)

Unless you're one of these people, you need a minimum of 2.5mcg (the RDA), but ideally you should take in 10mcg a day. For those with malabsorption of B12, which is very common in older people and occurs in two in five people in the UK[4], often 500mcg is required to normalise blood levels and bring the critical marker, homocysteine, down below 10mcmol/l (micromoles per litre). Homocysteine levels above this predict brain shrinkage leading to dementia.

The problem with plant sources of B12

Some foods contain 'false' B12, such as blue-green algae, for example spirulina, because it is in a form that is unable to bind to intrinsic factor. Hence, the list of nutritional ingredients of plant foods, unless fortified, might include B12 but whether or not this is *functional* B12 is debatable and should not be assumed.

Overall, it appears that when active B12 is present in plant foods, it is largely due to bacterial 'contamination', which could be more positively described as the plant having a symbiotic relationship with bacteria. This can occur, for example, in the cultivation of shiitake mushrooms where the logs that the mushrooms are grown on contain the bacteria, or in the open cultivation of algae such as chlorella and spirulina. Because the B12 in these instances is not *inherent* in the plant, but dependent on the *growing medium* or its symbiotic relationship with bacteria, these foods are a rather hit-and-miss source of B12. If the food is grown in a sterile environment, in contrast, it might not contain B12. Given this variability, it's hardly surprising that the Vegan Society advises that vegans supplement B12 and eat foods fortified with it.

Before we look at the best plant foods for B12 in the next section, given this caution, note that the evidence for their viability is largely derived from feeding people these foods and measuring their functional B12 status and the ability of these foods to correct a deficiency. (The best measure of B12 in the blood is called 'holotranscobalamin' or HoloTC, followed by methylmalonic acid or MMA, which goes up if deficient. A raised homocysteine level, meaning poor methylation, is also a very useful indicator. See

Resources for a home-test kit.) If you choose to rely on these foods for your B12, which I would not recommend, it is wise to check your B12 and homocysteine levels, and it is *essential* to do so if you're contemplating getting pregnant. If your B12 level or HoloTC is low (below 300pmol/l or 40pmol/l – picomoles per litre) or if your MMA is above 270nmol/l (nanomoles per litre) or your homocysteine is above 10mcmol/l then you are endangering your health.

Vitamin B12 in vegan foods

The plants that have been found to contain *some* B12 are various mushrooms, notably shiitake (as we saw above), blue-green algae, nori seaweed and sea buckthorn, which is a plant that grows close to the sea. Seaweed is algae that clings to rocks. Algae is divided into red algae, which grows in the sea, and blue-green algae, which grows in fresh water such as lakes.

Algae and seaweed – B12 in detail

Chlorella and spirulina are blue-green algae, whereas nori seaweed is red algae, eaten in China as *zicai*, Korea as *kim*, New Zealand as *karengo* and Wales as a traditional laverbread. Of all the plant foods, nori seems to be the best vegan food for B12[5]; however, you would have to eat a lot. To put this into context, an analysis of B12 in these different forms of nori found between 3mcg (in Welsh nori) and around 60mcg in Chinese and Korean nori per 100g.[6] A sheet of nori is 2.5g, so to achieve the RDA of 2.5mcg of the most B12-rich untoasted dried nori you would have to eat two sheets, but to achieve the ideal amount of 10mcg you would have to eat eight sheets a day.

Is this functional B12? It appears to have corrected B12 deficiency in animals; however, dried nori seems to be not as good as raw nori. In a study of female volunteers their B12 status got worse when given only *dried* nori (40g) but did not degenerate when given the equivalent amount of *raw* nori. On further analysis the researcher found that the B12 in the dried nori had converted the B12 into the 'false' form described above that cannot be efficiently absorbed.[7] Therefore, it's hard to rely on nori for B12. If some active B12 is present it is a result of bacterial contamination rather than inherent in the food itself.

The most commonly reported vegan foods for vitamin B12 are supplements or powders of chlorella or spirulina, farmed in freshwater vats and lakes. This is another rather hit-and-miss source. One analysis of 19 dried chlorella supplements found B12 levels varied from an insignificant less than 0.1mcg to 415mcg per 100g. A teaspoon is about 5g, so you would have to be eating the equivalent of 20 teaspoons to get these levels.

Chlorella grown in large open culture tanks were more likely to have more B12, and that is likely to come from bacterial contamination or the intended addition of B12 into the growing medium.[8] Chlorella itself does not require B12 to grow. That said, a study of 17 vegan or vegetarian adults given 9g, roughly two teaspoons, of chlorella powder for 60 days showed improvement in B12 status and a reduction in homocysteine, suggesting that the B12 in this chlorella was, at least, absorbable and functional.[9]

Spirulina fared worse, as one study found that 83 per cent of the B12 in the spirulina supplement they analysed was false B12.[10] Again, it is likely that any B12 in spirulina comes from bacteria in the growing medium rather than the algae itself; however, the news is not all bad for spirulina. An animal study found that B12-deficient animals fed spirulina for ten weeks did restore their B12 status[11]; however, previous studies have identified the B12 in spirulina as false B12,[12] which not only doesn't work but inhibits real B12 from working[13].

I would not rely on spirulina as a source of B12. Another algae, AFA algae (*Aphanizomenon flos-aquae*), like spirulina, is often claimed to provide B12, but it is also false B12.[14]

I'd be very wary of relying on chlorella as your only source of B12. If you do choose to use algae as a source of B12, and not directly supplement it, then I strongly recommend that you monitor your B12 level (see page 266).

The plus sides of seaweed and algae

Despite their drawbacks in relation to vitamin B12, seaweed and algae are excellent sources of other nutrients that can be lacking in a plant-based, or rather a land-based, diet, namely iodine and selenium. Iodine is essential for proper thyroid function, without which growth and brain development are stunted, whereas selenium is vital for healthy immunity. Both are found richly in seafood, including seaweed, and can be deficient in plant-based food grown on deficient soil, which means in landlocked regions and not grown organically. An easy way to increase seaweed in your diet is to eat, for example, dried nori seaweed sheets (see Resources) as a snack, and add it to salads as a garnish. Seaweed, in the UK, is certainly a food group that has been largely ignored, although it features heavily in Japanese food.

Mushrooms – an unreliable source of B12

Various mushrooms are touted as good sources of B12 but, in reality, the amount they provide is very low because, as we have seen, B12 is not produced by the mushroom but is present in the bacteria in the growing medium, and you don't know how much is *active* B12.

The two varieties that appear to have the most B12 are shiitake mushrooms and truffles. In the former the B12 is due to contamination from the logs they're grown on and the latter because of where they grow, namely underground and close to tree roots. Studies have measured around 5mcg in shiitake and 11mcg in truffles in a 100g dried portion. A cup (250ml by volume – or roughly a small handful) of fresh mushrooms is about 70g (about 7g dry mushrooms). This means that if you wanted to achieve the RDA (2.5mcg) you would need to be eating 50g of dried shiitake, or 500g of raw fresh shiitake. But, again, you don't know how much of this B12 is active. Although shiitake mushrooms do seem to have active B12, a study of Lion's Mane mushroom was found to have largely *inactive* B12.[15] The dirtier the mushrooms, the more likely they are to have B12 from bacteria in the soil or growing medium.

An illustration of this was a study measuring blood levels of B12 and homocysteine in ten vegans eating nori seaweed and wild mushrooms, and not taking supplements, versus supplementing vegans and vegetarians and meat eaters. The B12 status of the mushroom and seaweed-eating vegans was borderline and they also had low vitamin D levels (more of this on pages 139–141). The supplementing vegans were sufficient in all nutrients.[16]

Sea buckthorn – a questionable source of B12

Sea buckthorn (*Hippophae rhamnoides*) is a plant that grows by the sea. Its berries are ground into a powder that is sold as a supplement that is reported to contain vitamin B12 as well as many other nutrients, from vitamin C to omega-7 (a non-essential fat that acts as a good moisturiser – it's good for dry eyes – and has mild anti-inflammatory effects, as well as being helpful for improving insulin sensitivity). In one study, sea buckthorn was found to contain 37mcg of B12 in 100g.[17] That means that 10g, roughly two teaspoons, would provide 3.7mcg, which is more than the RDA. But, again, it is likely to be a result of symbiotic bacteria relating to where and how it grows rather than the plant itself, so the B12 might not be reliably available from all kinds of sea buckthorn or in consistently reasonable quantities. Sea buck-thorn oil is not likely to contain B12.

B12 fortified foods and supplements

As we have seen, although the RDA of B12 is 2.5mcg, an optimal level, which correlates with the healthiest levels of homocysteine, and consequently brain health – and it is also the level required for a healthy pregnancy – is around 10mcg a day. Many nutrition authorities have revised daily requirements to this level. B12 is stored in the liver, which is why people who can't absorb it are given monthly injections. This means it is not imperative that you get 10mcg *every day*, but rather an average of 70mcg *a week*.

Many vegan foods, especially those that replace a non-vegan source of B12, are fortified. This can include non-dairy milks, vegan yoghurts and cheeses, and vegan egg and meat substitutes. Some cereals are fortified, too. But do check. It's not a legal requirement for food producers. Nutritional and brewer's yeast don't contain B12, unless it is specifically added. Unless a product states that B12 is added, assume that it is not. B12 is light-sensitive, so keep the yeast in a dark cupboard or fridge and buy a yeast product in a light-proof container. Non-dairy yoghurts containing live bacteria, such as bifidobacteria, and some fermented foods containing bacteria, can also provide a little B12, but this is not declared on the label, as it's variable. It's worth checking the foods you buy and adding up how much you're getting. Often, fortified foods will provide around 1mcg per serving, so if in a day you eat three servings of fortified foods you'll be getting 3mcg. Let's take an example of a typical day:

2 cups of soya/oat/almond/coconut milk	2.0mcg
1 tsp (5g) of nutritional yeast with B12	1.0mcg
Live coconut yoghurt or a fermented food	approx. 0.5mcg
Total	**(about) 3.5mcg**

Supplementing vitamin B12

By far the easiest way to ensure you get enough B12 is to supplement 10mcg, or perhaps half this if you are consciously eating these fortified foods, plus nori and shiitake mushrooms or chlorella or spirulina. Nevertheless, since these are unreliable sources, the best route is to supplement 10mcg a day so that you know your needs are covered. Some people, around one in ten, are genetically less good at methylation, which is dependent on B12, and for these people supplementing 20mcg a day would be optimal and provide a good safety margin, since there's no way to know if you're that one in ten without genetic testing.

Vitamin B12 comes in different forms, all ending with -cobalamin. (It's a molecule attached to the mineral cobalt.) The most common is cyanocobalamin, which is cheap, synthetic and stable, and converts into the natural forms of B12, which are hydroxycobalamin, methylcobalamin and adenosylcobalamin. B12, in all these forms, is made from bacteria. There's an argument for having the natural forms, each of which does something slightly different in the body, but there's no strong evidence that one is vastly superior to another, except for those with inborn genetic abnormalities that might require one particular form of B12.

Most RDA-style multivitamins provide 2.5mcg, whereas optimum multivitamins usually provide 10mcg. Given that you'll also benefit from supplementing vitamin D (see page 141) it's best to choose a multivitamin that gives both 10mcg of B12 and 15mcg of vitamin D. (See Chapter 11 for guidance on supplementation.)

Best nutrition – the vegan dilemma

As a vegan you have made decisions about what you want to eat and wear as a way to protect the environment and animals, and for your health, but sometimes decisions can be difficult. Needless to say there are strong opinions, and views tend to get polarised. An example might be grazing animals. There are large parts of the world that are not suited to agriculture but they are good for grazing animals such as sheep. Apart from their meat, sheep provide wool, and the wool oil, lanolin, is a major source of vitamin D. Vitamin D can, however, be synthesised in a laboratory, but how is this done and is it the best way to produce this essential vitamin? We also 'synthesise' vitamin D in our skin in the presence of sunlight, but if we live in Europe, supplementing vitamin D is essential in the winter months. But which works better – animal, vegan or self-made vitamin D? I will be explaining all about this in the following section. What you ultimately choose to do is up to you.

Vitamin D – are you getting enough?

There are two forms of vitamin D – vitamin D2 is made in plants, notably mushrooms, whereas vitamin D3 is found in animal produce, with fish being the richest source, and it is also produced in the skin. Our main source of vitamin D is from sunlight acting on the skin, but you need to expose your arms and face for at least twenty minutes a day to make reasonable amounts. In fact, the vitamin D in mushrooms is made by exposing them to light, which then converts plant sterols into vitamin D.

D3 is somewhat more effective than D2; however, the synthetic D2 used in vegetarian supplements readily converts to D3 in the body, and even D3 in supplements, while not technically vegetarian, is mainly derived from the oil in wool, but can also be made from lichen as a vegan source.

Whatever the source of vitamin D, it has to convert into 25-hydroxyvitamin D, which acts more like a hormone than a vitamin. It used to be thought that vitamin D's only role was to fix calcium into bone, hence a deficiency results in rickets in children and osteoporosis in older adults. But in the last 20 years it has become clear that vitamin D has many other roles in the body, including controlling cell growth and inhibiting growth of cancer cells, boosting immunity, strengthening muscles and reducing inflammation. It also influences over 200 genes. It might also be helpful for preventing depression, especially in the winter, as well as reducing infections, the risk of numerous diseases including diabetes, heart disease and cancer, but also multiple sclerosis and other auto-immune and neurological diseases such as dementia and Parkinson's. In short, it's a no-brainer to keep your vitamin D level close to optimal.

Many people, especially vegans, don't get enough vitamin D, so much so that it is now recognised that everyone living in the far northern (and southern) hemisphere, where the angle of the sun in the winter is insufficient to make much vitamin D, and the cold climate is not conducive to exposing naked skin to sunlight, needs to supplement this versatile vitamin. On the other hand, if you live in sunnier climes and spend lots of time outdoors, you might just make enough from the synthesis of vitamin D acting on cholesterol in the skin. The body stores vitamin D, so if you spend a couple of weeks in the sun in the winter months that too might see you through.

Due to these variables it is ideal to know your vitamin D status by measuring your blood level of 25-hydroxyvitamin D. The level you're aiming for is 75nmol/l. Below 50nmol/l is considered inadequate. Fortunately, this is one inexpensive test that many GPs are willing to do. If not, you can get relatively inexpensive home test kits (see Resources). If your level is low, it's best to supplement 25mcg a day (1,000iu) and recheck that you've achieved a level of 75nmol/l or more.

How much do you need to take in to get your blood level up to 75nmol/l? A review of studies concludes that an intake of 20mcg (800iu) of vitamin D per day for all adults might bring 97 per cent of the population to a level of at least 50nmol/l and about 50 per cent up to 75nmol/l. This level optimises both disease prevention and bone health.[18]

Alternatively, supplementing 15mcg (600iu) a day, assuming you get some from sunlight and fortified foods, should keep you close to optimum. The current NHS recommendation in the UK is 10mcg, but the EU and US recommended intake has been increased to 15mcg a day. I consider a total intake of 30mcg to be closer to the optimum level. Thirty minutes of sun exposure a day might provide you with the equivalent of 10mcg.

In terms of dietary intake, what you'll achieve from a vegan diet is questionable, since only mushrooms that have been purposely exposed to light or UV radiation, and fortified foods, will give you any vitamin D. It is likely that vitamin D-enriched mushrooms will become increasingly available, which could provide 10mcg per 100g serving.[19] You can buy mushrooms and expose them to sunlight, or a UV lamp, and make your own. But even so it's hard to know how much you'll be getting.

Non-dairy milks are also often fortified with vitamin D, usually giving 1.5mcg per serving. If you have one or two glasses of these, plus a serving of mushrooms, and you spend 30 minutes a day outdoors and also supplement 15mcg you'll be in the optimum zone.

If you spend little time outdoors and/or you don't eat these kinds of foods, I'd recommend you supplement 25mcg a day, which is 1,000iu. This amount is also probably ideal in the winter months if you live far away from the equator. Many supplements, including drops, come in 25mcg doses. The Vegan Society recommends a supplement providing 20mcg a day.

Also, since vitamin D is stored in the body, it is not necessary to take it every day. Studies show that supplementing, for example, 25mcg × 7 = 175mcg, once a week is equally effective in raising blood levels.

Your quick guide to vitamins B12 and D

The two vitamins that are hard, or virtually impossible, to obtain in optimal amounts from a vegan diet are vitamins B12 and D.

- Dietary sources of B12, namely nori seaweed, chlorella and sea buckthorn are variable and unreliable as sources of vitamin B12.
- Hence it is best to supplement 10mcg of B12 a day and/or eat B12 fortified foods that provide this amount, or supplement the difference.
- The only vegan food source of vitamin D is sunlight- or UV light-exposed mushrooms, which should therefore state their enriched vitamin D content on the packet.
- Make a point of getting outdoors for at least 30 minutes a day. The more skin you expose to the sun, the more vitamin D you will make.
- Supplement between 15mcg and 25mcg of vitamin D, the higher level being more suitable either in the winter or for those who do not get daily sun exposure, and for all those living in the far northern or far southern hemisphere in the winter months when the angle of the sun is insufficient, and the weather is not conducive to exposing the skin, and hence making vitamin D in the skin.
- See Resources for a list of suggested supplements.

Chapter 9

The Importance of Minerals

In previous chapters we have looked at the amount of macro-nutrients – protein, fat and carbohydrate – that the body needs to function, as well the vital role that vitamins play in sustaining us and promoting optimum health. In this chapter, I examine the role of minerals. All the elements that make up our body are essential for health. We might be made up mostly of oxygen, carbon, hydrogen and nitrogen (over 90 per cent) but if you cast your mind back to biology lessons at school you'll remember the periodic table of elements and the fact that we are made up of many other elements, some in miniscule amounts, from iron to zinc.

In the body, these minerals are mainly used to regulate and balance our body chemistry; the exceptions are calcium, phosphorus and magnesium, which are the major constituents of bone. Sulphur is another, but it is largely ignored because it's a component of many proteins, so if you're not lacking protein you're unlikely to be lacking sulphur. These four, plus sodium and potassium, which control both the water balance and electrical signalling in the body, along with calcium and magnesium, are called macro-minerals because we need relatively large amounts each day (300–3,000mg). The remaining elements are called trace minerals because we need only traces each day (30mg–30mcg). But all these minerals are required in tiny amounts compared to carbon, hydrogen and oxygen. For example, a 63.5kg (10 stone) man needs 400g of carbohydrate a day but only 40mcg of chromium, which is less than a millionth of the amount. Yet chromium is no less important.

The main minerals to be mindful of

Although we need all the minerals mentioned above in order to be healthy, there are some that vegans need to be particularly aware of, not because you cannot get them from a plant-based diet, but because you need to be mindful about what you eat in order to achieve enough.

The most important in this respect are iron, iodine, selenium, calcium, magnesium and zinc. The last two are not more deficient in a vegan diet than in an omnivorous one; they are just the most commonly deficient in everyone's diet, and the most important for health. Selenium and iodine are found in the richest quantities in seafood, hence seaweed is an excellent source of both these minerals. Iron, like zinc, is abundant in 'seed' foods, including beans, lentils, nuts and seeds, so it can be well supplied in a healthy vegan diet. The iron found in plant-based foods is not as bioavailable as that found in meat, called haem iron, but it can be made more bioavailable (how to do this is explained on page 150). Calcium, although found richly in dairy products, is also in plentiful supply in seed foods, such as almonds, and many nut milks. Calcium is no more bioavailable from dairy milk than plants, as long as you have sufficient vitamin D. Magnesium is abundant in a healthy vegan diet and of great importance to health.

Let's explore these minerals in some detail because, if you eat the appropriate foods to get enough of these, you'll also achieve an optimal amount of the other essential minerals, namely potassium, sodium, manganese, copper and chromium.

Calcium – the bone builder

Nearly 1.3kg (3lb) of your body weight is calcium, and 99 per cent of this is in your bones and teeth. Calcium is needed to provide the rigid structure of the skeleton. It is particularly important in childhood when bones are growing, and also in the elderly because the ability to absorb calcium becomes impaired with age. The remaining 10g or so of calcium is found in the nerves, muscles and blood. Working together with magnesium, calcium is needed to enable nerves and muscles to 'fire'. It also assists the blood to clot and helps to maintain the right acid–alkaline balance.

The average Western diet provides, on average, about 900mg. That's more than the RDA for calcium, which ranges from 700mg for girls and adults to 1,000mg for teenage boys and 1,250mg for mothers when breast-feeding. Most of it comes from milk and cheese, which are poor sources; however, vegetables, pulses, nuts, whole grains and water provide significant quantities of both calcium and magnesium, and it is likely that our ancestors relied on these foods for their calcium, since they weren't milking buffaloes.

What has emerged in recent years is that too much calcium can be a problem, especially in the absence of magnesium, which has a push-me-pull-you effect.

Magnesium, for example, relaxes arterial muscles thereby lowering blood pressure, whereas calcium does the opposite. Since there's no money to be made out of non-patentable magnesium, there's a class of drugs for hypertension that block the calcium channel into arterial muscle cells, increasing the relative magnesium–calcium ratio, and thus lowering blood pressure. It's a long way round, with side effects, but these calcium channel-blocker drugs do lower blood pressure.

Too much calcium in your bloodstream can also become incorporated into arterial plaques and, as a result, measuring coronary artery calcium (CAC) is a reasonably reliable indicator of risk of heart disease.

I never believed the linear argument that, since bones contain calcium and milk contains calcium, we need to drink lots of milk for healthy bones. This idea was further magnified by the medical profession buying into the idea that as post-menopausal women started to develop thinning bones they would need even more calcium. Studies giving calcium supplements to post-menopausal women have been largely unsuccessful, however. On the other hand, studies where vitamin D was given, which is the critical factor that drives calcium into bone, *have* been successful. Although some studies giving combined calcium with vitamin D have been successful, I believe it is largely to do with vitamin D's positive effect, and not the extra calcium. I say this because areas that have low calcium intake but good sunlight exposure and vitamin D status, such as equatorial Africa, have extremely low incidence of osteoporosis and fractures.

The best vegan food sources of calcium

Food	Milligrams of calcium
100g calcium-set firm tofu	350mg
2 slices of calcium-fortified bread	242mg
200ml calcium-fortified nut milk	240mg
125ml calcium-fortified soya yoghurt	150mg
2 tbsp tahini	128mg

Food	Milligrams of calcium
2 cups (120g/4¼oz) broccoli	124mg
80g cooked kale	120mg
30g almonds	72mg
1 tbsp chia seeds	69mg
1 tbsp almond butter	55mg

Calcium absorption by the body

The ability of the body to use the calcium from food depends not only on how much calcium is consumed but also on its ability to be absorbed. The amount absorbed depends on the type of food it comes from, but it is normally about 20–30 per cent. For kale it is 40 per cent and for watercress it's 27 per cent, but spinach, high in oxalic acid, is only 5 per cent. Whole milk, as a comparison, is 26 per cent. Cooking spinach, which helps lessen the oxalic acid level, improves calcium absorption.

The calcium balance of the body is *improved* where there are adequate levels of vitamin D and by weight-bearing exercise. The balance is made *worse* by vitamin D deficiency, consumption of alcohol, coffee and tea or a lack of hydrochloric acid produced in the stomach. The presence of naturally occurring chemicals called phytates, which are found in grains, also interferes with absorption, as do oxalates in spinach and rhubarb. Excessive protein consumption also causes a loss of calcium from the bones, but that's not going to happen on a vegan diet.

Given that you might be taking in a bit less calcium, perhaps 500–700mg on a vegan diet, and some of this will be from foods high in phytates, I would recommend supplementing about 300mg calcium a day, but not more than this unless you are breast-feeding, at which time 500mg might be appropriate.

Symptoms of deficiency include muscle cramps, tremors or spasms, insomnia, nervousness, joint pain, osteoarthritis, tooth decay and high blood pressure. Only severe deficiency causes osteoporosis.

Magnesium drives over 300 enzymes

The mineral magnesium works with calcium in maintaining bone density, and nerve and muscle impulses. But it also has many other roles in the body as a co-factor for over 300 enzymes, not least of which are those involved in making energy from food. It helps to stabilise blood sugar levels and is therefore very important for diabetics. It is also involved in protein synthesis and is essential for the production of certain hormones and in balancing out mood. Magnesium, therefore, helps reduce the severity of pre-menstrual syndrome, and also breast tenderness and water retention. It's very important for brain function, too, reducing anxiety. Magnesium is depleted by stress.

The average diet is relatively high in calcium but deficient in magnesium, because milk, a major source of calcium for non-vegans, is not a very good source of magnesium. Most people are taking in about 270mg of magnesium, but at least 500mg is preferable. Both minerals are present in green leafy vegetables, nuts and seeds. Magnesium is a vital component of chlorophyll, which gives plants their green colour and is therefore present in all green vegetables; however, only a small proportion of the magnesium within plants is in the form of chlorophyll.

There's also lots of magnesium in seeds and nuts. The best seeds are sesame and chia, followed by sunflower and pumpkin, while the best nuts are almonds and cashew nuts. Fifty grams of chia seeds provide 165mg of magnesium, the ideal daily intake being between 300mg and 500mg. Another great food for magnesium is wheatgerm.

The best vegan food sources of magnesium

100g of food	Milligrams of magnesium
Wheatgerm	490mg
Sesame seeds	351mg
Chia seeds	330mg
Sunflower seeds	325mg
Almonds	270mg
Cashew nuts	267mg
Pumpkin seeds	262mg
Brewer's yeast	231mg
Buckwheat flour	229mg
Brazil nuts	225mg
Peanuts	175mg
Pecan nuts	142mg
Cooked beans	37mg

I supplement at least 150mg of magnesium every day, but I recommend twice this for anyone with cardiovascular concerns, such as high blood pressure, or those suffering from mental-health issues, anxiety, stress or insomnia. A lack of magnesium is strongly associated with cardiovascular disease and high blood pressure, as well as diabetes.

Iron – the oxygen carrier

Iron is a vital component of haemoglobin in the blood, which transports oxygen and carbon dioxide to and from cells. Sixty per cent of the iron within us is in the form of red pigment or haem. This is the form present in meat, and it is much more readily absorbed than the non-haem iron present in non-meat food sources. Non-haem iron occurs in the oxidised or ferric state in food, and not until it is reduced to the ferrous state (for example, by vitamin C) during digestion can it be absorbed. Vegan food sources of iron such as beans, lentils, nuts and seeds contain as much as, if not more than, meat and, although not so well absorbed, if you take a vitamin C supplement with a meal containing these foods you could easily double your absorption.

Men need about 10–15mg a day and menstruating women 15–20mg. Very few women get close to this amount, however. The average intake of women in the UK is 10mg. More than half of all teenage girls achieve less than half this amount, as do a third of women. What, then, do you need to eat?

In most tables showing the nutrients in foods, there's a bit of a cheat going on that falsely favours meat. Foods are listed in the order of how much of the nutrient there is per 100g. We don't eat by weight, however. In other words, you could eat a lot more weight of broccoli than meat or cheese before you were full. That feeling-full criterion is closer to the calories in the food than the weight in grams. Below I list the foods in the order of those with the most iron per calorie, then added how much you'd get if you ate 100g.

The best vegan food sources of iron

100g of food	Milligrams of iron
Pumpkin seeds	11.2mg
Parsley	6.2mg
Almonds	4.7mg
Prunes	3.9mg
Cashew nuts	3.6mg
Raisins	3.5mg
Brazil nuts	3.4mg
Walnuts	3.1mg
Dates	3.0mg
Cooked dried beans	2.7mg
Red lentils	2.4mg
Sesame seeds	2.4mg
Pecan nuts	2.4mg

Although 100g is a lot of seeds or nuts to eat in one go, 50g is achievable in a meal, and 100g of nuts, seeds, beans or lentils is certainly achievable across one day, giving you something in the region of 6mg of iron. That alone is not enough, however, and that's why I recommend supplementing 10mg, which is what I take daily. For menstruating women, it is wise to achieve 15mg a day. Post-menopause, 10mg a day in total is probably enough.

The symptoms of iron deficiency include pale skin, a sore tongue, fatigue or listlessness, a loss of appetite, and nausea. Anaemia is clinically diagnosed by checking haemoglobin levels in the blood; however, symptoms of anaemia can also be caused by a lack of vitamin B12 or folic acid. Iron-deficiency anaemia is most likely to occur in women, especially during pregnancy. Since iron is an antagonist to zinc, increasing the requirement for zinc, supplements containing more than 30mg of iron (over twice the RDA), should not be taken without ensuring that enough zinc is also being consumed. Although iron supplements are often given in doses above 50mg, there is little evidence that this is more effective than lower doses in raising haemoglobin levels.

Zinc

A large part of the vegetarian population is at risk of being zinc deficient, according to the conclusion of reviews of all studies to date[1] and the difference is greater when comparing pregnant vegan or vegetarian women with meat eaters[2]. This is a worry because zinc is one of the most commonly deficient minerals of all. Also, it is especially important in pregnancy, since zinc is essential for all growth. There is a strong correlation between low birth weight and zinc deficiency, so much so that any child born weighing below 13.13kg (6lb 14oz) is suspected of having sub-optimal levels of zinc.

This is easily avoidable, however, because zinc is found richly in nuts, seeds, beans, lentils and basically anything that grows when you plant it. But, as with iron, vegans have to either consciously eat a lot of these foods or supplement zinc – ideally both.

The best vegan food sources of zinc

100g of food	Milligrams of zinc
Ginger root	6.8mg
Pecan nuts	4.5mg
Dry split peas	4.2mg

100g of food	Milligrams of zinc
Green peas	1.6mg
Turnips	1.2mg
Brazil nuts	4.2mg
Wholewheat grains	3.2mg
Rye	3.2mg
Oats	3.2mg
Peanuts	3.2mg
Almonds	3.1mg

You need at least 10mg (the RDA), but many studies show better mental health and immune function with higher intakes up to 20mg a day. I supplement 15mg a day, along with 10mg in my daily multivitamin and mineral.

With half the population eating less than half the RDA, few people get enough from their diet. Deficiency symptoms include white marks on the nails, a lack of appetite or a lack of appetite control, pallor, infertility, lack of resistance to infection, poor growth (including hair growth), poor skin (including acne, dermatitis and stretch marks), plus mental and emotional problems.

Zinc deficiency plays a role in nearly every major disease, including diabetes and cancer. Zinc is needed to make insulin, to boost the immune system and to make the antioxidant enzyme SOD (superoxide dismutase), a key player in keeping you young and healthy. It is also required to make prostaglandins from essential fats. These hormone-like substances help to balance hormones and to control inflammation and the stickiness of the blood. Sucking zinc lozenges helps to shorten the duration of a cold.

Zinc's main role is the protection and repair of DNA, and for this reason it is found in higher levels in animals and fish than in plants (because animals have higher levels of DNA). A vegan diet, therefore, tends to be low in zinc, and phytates in grains also make it less easy to absorb. Stress, smoking and alcohol deplete it, as does frequent sex, at least for men, since semen contains very high concentrations of zinc. That's why oysters are popularly said to be aphrodisiacs. They are also the highest dietary source of zinc, providing about 15mg per oyster, and for both men and women zinc is essential for fertility. There are plenty of vege-burgers and vege-sausages but I've never seen a zinc-enriched vege-oyster!

Even if you're a fan of eating lots of nuts, seeds and beans, I'd recommend you cover your bases by supplementing at least 10mg of zinc a day.

Selenium and iodine – the sea minerals

Selenium and iodine are two minerals that you don't need much of but without which serious mental and physical health problems occur. Although you need 500mg of magnesium daily, you need only 50mcg of selenium and 150mcg of iodine. One thousand micrograms (mcg) is a milligram (mg), so you need 10,000 times more magnesium than selenium.

Both selenium and iodine are found abundantly in the sea and therefore in all seafood, including seaweed. Certain geographic areas far from the sea throughout the planet's evolution have low selenium and/or iodine levels, thus leading to deficiency. Areas that were under the sea in the past, but now are not, can have particularly high levels.

One good example of this is the Wash in Suffolk, which has the highest proportion of people living to over 100 in the UK. Selenium is vital for the immune system to work properly, and a lack of it is associated with a high risk of infections and certain cancers. Wherever iodine soil levels are low there is a high incidence of goitre, a thyroid disease that leads to cretinism, because a child's brain cannot develop without iodine, which is essential for the thyroid to work.

Selenium – a tiny mineral with a big kick

The mineral selenium works with glutathione, forming a dynamic duo in the critical antioxidant enzyme called glutathione peroxidase, sometimes abbreviated to GPX. It is a trace element, which means you need very little. The amount you and I need on a daily basis is probably 50mcg, up to a maximum of 200mcg when under viral attack. It's also one of the most toxic minerals. You certainly don't want more than 500mcg.

There's even a theory that low selenium levels in the diet of Asian bats, and in people in Hubei, might have allowed the Covid-19 virus to develop, since selenium not only inhibits viral replication but appears to block its ability to mutate.[3]

Deficiency of this mineral was first discovered in China as the cause of Keshan disease, a type of heart disease prevalent in areas in which the soil is deficient in selenium. It has since been associated with another regional disease, this time in Russia, involving joint degeneration. Perhaps the most significant finding is selenium's association with a low risk of certain kinds of cancer.

As mentioned above, selenium is the vital constituent of the antioxidant enzyme glutathione peroxidase. A tenfold increase in dietary selenium causes a doubling of the quantity of this enzyme in the body. Since many oxides are cancer producing, and since cancer cells destroy other cells by releasing oxides, it is likely to be selenium's role in glutathione peroxidase production that gives it protective properties against cancer and premature ageing. It might also be essential for the thyroid gland, which controls the body's rate of metabolism. Selenium is found predominantly in whole foods, particularly seafood, including seaweed, and sesame seeds and nuts. If you grind the seeds, the nutrients become more readily available. But it does depend entirely on the soil level where the plant grows. One prevailing myth is that Brazil nuts are a rich source of selenium, but some Brazil nuts contain none. Unfortunately, you can't guarantee your intake by eating nuts. Seaweed, on the other hand, will always be a reliable source of both selenium and iodine.

Normally, you would aim for an intake of 50–70mcg, perhaps 100mcg as an optimum. During an infection, however, it would be wise to increase your selenium intake to 200mcg. I generally assume that I'll eat 50mcg from my wholefood diet, which includes seaweed (I like nori seaweed crisps – see Resources) so I supplement an additional 30mcg in my daily multivitamin; however, the antioxidant supplement I take provides another 50mcg. Most antioxidant formulas do. That might give me a little over 100mcg. Selenium is one mineral you don't want to take too much of, however, as mentioned earlier. It becomes toxic certainly above 500mcg, causing nausea, vomiting, nail discoloration and brittleness, hair loss, fatigue and irritability.

Iodine – your thyroid's best friend

The thyroid gland, at the base of your throat, controls the accelerator of your metabolism. It produces a hormone, thyroxine, which speeds up the production of energy. Too much thyroxine and you end up manic, but too little, which is far more common, and you feel tired all the time, with sluggish digestion, inability to control your temperature, thus easily feeling too hot or too cold, and you gain weight. An underactive thyroid is experienced by at least one in 50 women in the UK, and it's six times more common in women than men.

Iodine is needed to make thyroxine, so iodine deficiency is one cause of an underactive thyroid. If a woman is iodine deficient in pregnancy the foetal brain cannot develop properly, therefore it is absolutely essential to have enough during pregnancy.[4] Low iodine in pregnancy, and in infants, is associated with lower IQ and mental health problems such as ADHD in children. Being such a tiny trace element, with levels in plants entirely dependent upon the soil they grow in, it is worth either supplementing, or eating iodine-fortified foods or seaweed. That one sheet of dried nori seaweed can cover two bases – providing selenium and iodine.

Iodine is often added to table salt, although genuine sea salt will also provide some. A good multivitamin will include some iodine, perhaps 30mcg. One of Clearspring's Seaveg Crispies (my favourite seaweed snack) provides 57mcg. Two of these a day, plus iodine in a multivitamin, achieves the optimal intake of 150mcg, which is especially wise during pregnancy and breast-feeding. Otherwise 50–100mcg a day is probably optimal.

Your quick guide to important minerals

Many people fall short of essential minerals unless they eat a wholefood diet.

- The most commonly deficient minerals generally are zinc and magnesium.
- On a vegan diet it is easier to be deficient in iron, zinc, selenium and iodine.
- Zinc and iron are found richly in nuts, seeds, beans and lentils.
- Iron absorption is helped by vitamin C.
- Selenium and iodine are found in seaweed.
- It is wise to supplement a multivitamin and mineral providing about 10mg of both zinc and iron, plus 30–50mcg of selenium and iodine.

- Be mindful of your calcium intake. It is found richly in seeds, nuts and nut milks and greens. Do not supplement more than 300mg of calcium, and ideally with at least 150mg of magnesium, unless pregnant or breast-feeding.
- See Resources for a list of suggested supplements.

Part 3

Healthy Vegan Recipes and Supplements

This is the practical section that shows you how to choose the right foods and make delicious meals and snacks that will apply the principles explained in the book.

You'll also find practical guidance on the supplements that have been discussed in earlier chapters.

Chapter 10

Vegan Recipes

The recipes are designed to be healthy, delicious and simple – and are GL-calculated to allow you to plan your meals and avoid see-sawing blood sugar levels. The GL of each recipe has been calculated per serving, but note that the recipes vary in how many they serve, as some are simple breakfasts, others are perfect for two for lunch and some are good cooked in bulk for a family, eaten as leftovers or frozen.

Breakfasts

Wild Mushrooms on Toast

Strongly flavoured wild mushrooms are quite delicious served simply, on toast. You might like to add some lightly wilted spinach to increase your green leafy veg quota, and perhaps have some soya yoghurt or a handful of nuts or pumpkin seeds in addition to this dish to boost the protein content. This recipe serves two, as wild mushrooms are a nice weekend breakfast or brunch to share.

Serves 2
GL per serving: 10

25g coconut oil, plus a little melted oil for drizzling
150g wild mushrooms (or white, button or chestnut mushrooms), brushed or wiped
2 slices wholegrain bread
salt and freshly ground black pepper
flat-leaf parsley sprig or finely chopped chives, to garnish

1. Heat the oil in a frying pan over a medium heat, then fry the mushrooms until soft. Toast the bread while the mushrooms are cooking.
2. Season to taste and drain the excess water from the mushrooms.
3. Drizzle some coconut oil over the toast and spoon the mushrooms on top. Garnish with the parsley and serve.

Porridge with Almonds and Goji Berries

Flaked almonds add flavour and more protein to a sustaining bowl of porridge. If goji berries aren't available, try chopped dried apricots instead (organic or unsulfured apricots are best).

Serves 1
GL per serving: 3

4 tbsp porridge oats
water or plant-based milk, or a 50:50 blend, in a ratio of 2 parts liquid to 1 part oats
2 tsp–1 tbsp goji berries, to taste
1 tbsp flaked almonds

1. Put the oats in a small pan. Add double the amount of water, milk or a blend of both.
2. Bring to a gentle simmer and allow to bubble and thicken for a few minutes, until the oats have swollen.
3. Pour into a bowl, then sprinkle with goji berries and almonds before serving.

Apple and Hazelnut Granola

Dried apple lends a natural sweetness to this recipe, while using oats and xylitol instead of sugar make it a much lower GL than most granolas. Enjoy served with fresh berries and soya or coconut yoghurt.

Serves 4
GL per serving: 4

2 tbsp coconut oil
150g whole oat flakes, or a blend of oat and barley flakes
3 tbsp hazelnut butter
3 tbsp hazelnuts with skins, chopped
1 tbsp milled chia seeds or ground flaxseed
1 tbsp wheatgerm, or seeds if you prefer it to be wheat-free
2 tbsp finely chopped dried apple slices, or to taste
1 tbsp xylitol
2 tsp ground mixed spice, or to taste

1. Melt the oil in a frying pan over a medium heat, then add the oats and stir to coat evenly. Cook for 1 minute or until slightly crisp.
2. Mix in the hazelnut butter as best as you can to coat evenly.
3. Stir in the remaining ingredients. Taste and adjust the flavour by adding more sweetness or spice as preferred. Leave to cool, then store in an airtight container for instant breakfasts.

Bircher Muesli

This meltingly soft, slightly chewy mixture of fruity goodness is quite delicious. The dried apple and the bursts of blueberry provide sweetness, but if you prefer a little more, you could add ½ tsp xylitol.

Serves 1
GL per serving: 6

4 tbsp oat flakes
1 tbsp wheatgerm, or ground almonds if you prefer it wheat-free
1 tbsp ground almonds, or flaked for a coarser texture
1 tbsp pumpkin seeds, or another type of seed or nut
1 tsp ground cinnamon, or to taste
10g, or about 1 heaped tbsp, finely chopped dried apple rings
3 tbsp frozen or fresh blueberries, or to taste
150ml plant-based milk, or to taste

1. Put the oats in a bowl. Mix in the wheatgerm, almonds, seeds and cinnamon.
2. Add the apples and blueberries and pour in the milk. Stir to coat everything, then cover.
3. Chill in the fridge for an hour to let the oats swell and soften, or make it the night before, ready for breakfast the next morning. You can always add more sweetness, cinnamon, berries or milk to change the flavour or consistency if you like.

Chia Pancakes with Pear Compote

Unlike traditional pancakes, which use processed white flour, these little pancakes are made with oats and chia seeds. The texture is a little coarser, but they are just as moreish and much healthier. This recipe makes enough for four people, but the pancakes keep well for 2 days in the fridge or can be frozen.

Serves 4 (makes 8 pancakes)
GL per serving: 6

1 tbsp ground flaxseed
45g oats
45g milled chia seeds
35g xylitol
225ml plant-based milk, such as almond
virgin rapeseed oil for frying

Pear compote:
2 large pears, cored and diced
1 tsp ground mixed spice or cinnamon, or to taste
xylitol to taste (optional)

1. Put the flaxseed in a bowl and add 3 tablespoons of cold water.
   Leave to soak for 20 minutes.
2. To make the pear compote, put the pears in a small pan with a
   tiny dash of water and the spice. Bring to a simmer, then cover
   and leave to cook for 5 minutes or until just softened. Taste and
   add more spice if you like. You could sweeten the mixture with a
   little xylitol if you feel it needs it. Set aside, with the lid on, while
   you make the pancakes.
3. Grind the oats with the chia seeds into as fine a flour as you can.
   If your food processor leaves the mixture coarse, try a hand
   blender to achieve a smoother finish. Mix the xylitol into the flour.
4. Mix the ground flaxseed and milk together and stir into the flour
   mixture to form a smooth batter. The chia absorbs liquid, so it
   will thicken more than a standard pancake batter.
5. Heat 1–2 tablespoons of oil in a large frying pan, then spoon in
   tablespoonfuls of the batter, spreading each out into a rough
   circle and taking care not to let them touch. Do this in batches
   and cook each pancake for 1–2 minutes on each side, or until
   golden and firmed up, before turning over. Press down in the pan

to flatten and help them cook. Put the cooked pancakes onto a warmed plate as they cook, and cover with a tea towel to keep them warm. Serve with the fruit.

Tip
The pancakes can be frozen.

Blueberry and Banana Smoothie

In this smoothie the fruit provides energy, the berries contain vitamins and antioxidants, the soya yoghurt provides protein and the seeds contain essential fats, as well as protein and zinc. The seeds add texture, but if you prefer a smooth consistency, grind them in a coffee-bean grinder or food processor first.

Serves 4
GL per serving: 12

600g blueberries
2 bananas, roughly chopped
180ml soya yoghurt
4 tbsp pumpkin or sunflower seeds
a little soya milk, juice or water if needed

1. Put the blueberries, bananas, yoghurt and seeds in a blender or food processor and whiz until smooth.
2. Check the consistency, and if you think it needs it, add a small amount of liquid to make the smoothie easier to drink.

Oat Crunch Yoghurt Pots

Pear and cinnamon are perfect flavour partners. This is a complete breakfast containing protein from the nuts and yoghurt to combine with the oats and will see you through to lunch.

Serves 4
GL per serving: 10

4 pears, cored and roughly chopped
½–1 tsp ground cinnamon, to taste
1 tbsp coconut oil or light olive oil
1 tbsp xylitol
50g whole oat flakes
1 tbsp flaked almonds
1 tbsp ground almonds
1 tbsp roughly chopped macadamia nuts, hazelnuts or any other
    raw, unsalted nuts
1 tbsp pumpkin seeds
400g soya yoghurt

1. Put the pears and a dash of water in a saucepan, cover and
   simmer for 3–5 minutes or until fairly soft. Add a little cinnamon
   to taste. Set aside to cool.
2. Make the topping by gently heating the oil in a frying pan over
   a medium heat. Add the xylitol, oats, nuts and seeds, and
   stir for 2 minutes or so to allow the oats to toast slightly. Set
   aside to cool.
3. Divide the pears between four shallow glasses or bowls, cover
   with the yoghurt and top with the nut mixture.

Chocolate and Goji Granola

This chewy, chocolatey granola might seem far too decadent for
breakfast but in fact it's a cunningly disguised healthy option. It is
packed with seeds to provide omega-3 and -6 essential fats, as well
as vitamin C and amino acids from the goji. The cacao powder adds
a rich, chocolate flavour, but with none of the added fat and sugar of
processed chocolate.

Serves 4
GL per serving: 10

3 tbsp coconut oil or light olive oil
150g whole oat flakes
3 tbsp tahini
3 tbsp pumpkin seeds
3 tbsp sunflower seeds
3 tbsp sesame seeds
3 tbsp poppy seeds
3 tbsp desiccated coconut
3 tbsp goji berries
4 tsp xylitol or to taste
1 tsp ground cinnamon, or to taste
1 tsp ground ginger, or to taste
4 tbsp cacao powder, or cocoa powder, or to taste

1. Gently heat the oil in a frying pan over a medium heat. Add the oat flakes and stir to coat them with the oil. Mix in the tahini as best you can, trying to spread it around the oats fairly evenly.
2. Turn off the heat and stir in the remaining ingredients. Taste and adjust the flavour by adding more xylitol, cinnamon, ginger or cacao if necessary. Serve.

Tip
Can be made in advance and stored in an airtight container in the fridge for up to 1 week.

Superfruit Salad

You can vary the fruit used according to your taste and the season, but the following recipe is a fabulous summer fruit salad to top up vitamin C levels. The blended yoghurt and fruit make a delicious fresh topping for pouring over the fruit salad, while the seeds add protein and essential fats. This dish should be served straightaway, and is great for reminding guests or family that fruit is one of nature's best breakfasts.

Serves 4
GL per serving: 13

seeds of ½ pomegranate
150g strawberries, hulled and chopped
100g blueberries, diced
2 small bananas, thinly sliced
4 apricots or plums, or 2 peaches or nectarines, stoned and chopped
180ml soya or coconut yoghurt
100g fresh berries
a little xylitol or agave syrup, to taste (optional)
4 tbsp ground flaxseed
2 tbsp pumpkin seeds
2 tbsp sunflower seeds
2 tbsp wheatgerm

1. Put the pomegranate seeds into a large bowl and add the strawberries, blueberries, bananas and apricots. Mix together and then divide among four bowls.
2. Put the yoghurt in a bowl and stir in the other fresh berries. Sweeten to taste with the xylitol, if needed.
3. Pour the blended fruit yoghurt over the fruit salad and sprinkle the seeds and wheatgerm on top. Serve.

Banana Muffins

These muffins are very simple to make and are a far better option than the coffee-shop version, which is likely to be heavily sweetened and made from refined white flour. You can use oat, rice or almond milk, whichever you prefer. The sunflower seeds sprinkled on top provide crunch plus vitamin E and omega-6 fats. If you prefer, they could be replaced with pumpkin seeds (or omitted).

Makes 8
GL per muffin: 11

2 tbsp ground flaxseed
75g coconut oil or dairy-free margarine suitable for baking
50g xylitol
2 large bananas, roughly sliced
120ml oat, rice or almond milk
1 tsp vanilla extract
150g plain wholemeal flour
1 tsp baking powder
1 tsp bicarbonate of soda
50g dried mixed fruit or raisins
25g sunflower seeds

1. Put the flaxseed in a small bowl and add 90ml cold water. Leave to soak for 20 minutes.
2. Preheat the oven to 180°C/350°F/Gas 4. Grease eight muffin cases and put in a muffin tray or on a baking sheet.
3. In a large bowl, cream the coconut oil and xylitol together until soft and creamy.
4. Blend or mix in all the remaining ingredients, except for the dried fruit and seeds, until smooth. If you are doing this by hand, it is easier to mash the bananas separately.
5. Stir in the dried fruit and spoon two heaped tablespoons of the mixture into each of the muffin cases. Sprinkle the tops with sunflower seeds.
6. Bake for 25–30 minutes until the tops are starting to turn golden and are fairly firm to the touch, then leave on the tray for 5 minutes. Remove the muffins from the tray and put on a wire rack to cool completely. Store in an airtight container.

Tip
Suitable for freezing.

Snacks and light meals

Tamari Toasted Nuts

These are irresistibly tasty, yet high in protein and minerals and low in carbohydrate and saturated fat. Take them to work in a small sealed container, or serve as nibbles. You can make up to a week's worth of this snack and store them in an airtight container in the fridge.

Serves 2
GL per serving: 2

50g mixed nuts and seeds (such as Brazil nuts, pecan nuts, walnuts, almonds, pine nuts, pumpkin seeds, sesame seeds or sunflower seeds)
1 tbsp tamari or soy sauce

Preheat the oven to 200°C/400°F/Gas 6. Put the nuts and seeds on a baking tray, tip the soy sauce over them and shake around to coat thoroughly. Roast for 5 minutes, shaking the tray halfway through. Leave to cool.

Red Pepper and Cucumber Salsa

A zesty dollop of this will liven up vegan burgers. Raw vegetables are packed with vitamins and antioxidants, making this salsa super-healthy.

Serves 2
GL per serving: 2

1 red onion, chopped

4 cherry tomatoes, cut into small chunks

½ red pepper, deseeded and chopped

1 tbsp extra virgin olive oil

2 tsp finely chopped fresh flat-leaf parsley leaves

5cm chunk of cucumber, cut lengthways into quarters, then sliced horizontally into triangles

2 tsp deseeded and finely chopped red chilli

2 tsp lemon juice

freshly ground black pepper

Put all the ingredients in a bowl and mix together well. Serve.

Guacamole

Fresh chilli, garlic and spring onions give this version of the Mexican speciality a real kick. This recipe is easy to throw together in minutes. Serve with vegetable crudités.

Serves 2
GL per serving: 1

1 ripe avocado, roughly chopped

juice of ½ lime

2 garlic cloves, crushed

1 tbsp finely chopped fresh coriander leaves

4 spring onions, finely chopped

¼ mild chilli, deseeded

salt and freshly ground black pepper

Put all the ingredients in a bowl and mash together using a fork. Season to taste and serve.

Roasted Red Pepper Hummus

It's always worthwhile making your own hummus. In this recipe, the slightly smoky, sweet taste of roasted red peppers adds oomph. Hummus makes a healthy snack with vegetable crudités.

Serves 4
GL per serving: 2.5

400g can chickpeas, rinsed and drained
1 tbsp lemon juice
75g or 1 large roasted red pepper from the deli or a jar
2 garlic cloves, crushed
1 tsp ground cumin
1 tbsp tahini
1 tbsp chopped fresh flat-leaf parsley leaves
1 tbsp extra virgin olive oil
freshly ground black pepper

Put all the ingredients in a food processor and whiz until smooth. Serve.

Tip
You can double the quantities for this recipe and store it in the fridge for up to 3 days.

Pine Nut and Sun-Dried Pepper Hummus

This version of the classic Middle Eastern dip is given a Mediterranean flavour by the pine nuts and sun-dried peppers. For a light meal, serve it with salad and wholemeal bread or pitta.

Serves 2
GL per serving: 8

400g can chickpeas, drained and rinsed
juice of ½ lemon, or to taste
1 large garlic clove, crushed
1 tbsp tahini
75ml extra virgin olive oil, or to taste
1 tsp sea salt, or to taste
50g sun-dried or roasted peppers in olive oil, drained
2 tbsp pine nuts

1. Put the chickpeas into a food processor and add the lemon juice, garlic, tahini, oil (use more or less depending on the consistency preferred or use some of the drained oil from the sun-dried peppers) and salt. Whiz together until smooth and creamy.
2. Add the peppers and pine nuts, and blend again to combine – you can leave a slightly coarser texture if you prefer. Taste and adjust the seasoning and consistency by adding more lemon juice, oil or salt if you like. Serve.

Sun-Dried Tomato and Black Olive Pesto

The intense flavours of sun-dried tomatoes and olives are delicious with wholemeal pasta or mixed with chickpeas or borlotti beans and chopped fresh vegetables for a quick, substantial salad with a complete protein profile.

Serves 2 (makes 2 tbsp pesto)
GL per serving: 2

50g sun-dried tomato paste
50g pitted black olives
50g pine nuts
10g fresh flat-leaf parsley leaves
25g fresh basil leaves
2 garlic cloves, crushed

2 tsp lemon juice
I tbsp extra virgin olive oil
freshly ground black pepper

Put all the ingredients in a small food processor or mini chopper and blend until fairly smooth. Serve.

Pumpkin Seed Pesto

It's wonderful when something that tastes this amazing is also really good for you – pumpkin seed butter is rich in omega-3s. Stir this dark-green pesto through soup or pasta, spread it on your favourite bread or add it to bean or lentil salads.

Serves 2 (makes 2 tbsp pesto)
GL per serving: I

25g pumpkin seeds
40g pumpkin seed butter
I0g fresh flat-leaf parsley leaves
I0g fresh basil leaves
I garlic clove, crushed
I tsp lemon juice
½ tbsp extra virgin olive oil

1. Put the pumpkin seeds in a food processor or nut mill and grind until roughly chopped.
2. Put the pumpkin seed butter in a small blender or food processor and add the chopped pumpkin seeds, herbs, garlic and lemon juice. Blitz until the mixture is well combined.
3. Add the oil and mix until the pesto is an even consistency. Serve.

Aubergine Pâté

The aubergine and borlotti beans give a lovely flavour to this delicious pâté, which is rich in antioxidants from the onion, garlic and tomato purée. Serve with a low-carb bread or oatcakes for a tasty and healthy snack.

Serves 2
GL per serving: 5

1 tsp coconut oil or light olive oil
1 garlic clove, crushed
1 red onion, chopped
¼ aubergine, cubed
1 tbsp tomato purée
½ can borlotti beans, rinsed and drained
½ tsp mixed dried herbs
1 tsp vegetable bouillon powder
freshly ground black pepper

1. Heat the oil in a saucepan over a medium heat and cook the garlic for 30 seconds, then add the onion and cook for 5 minutes or until softened.
2. Add the aubergine and cook for 10 minutes or until it browns and softens.
3. Add the tomato purée, beans, dried herbs and bouillon powder, and stir together, then season with black pepper to taste.
4. Put the mixture in a food processor and blitz until it is fairly smooth. Serve.

Wild Rice, Artichoke and Aduki Bean Salad

Aduki beans are a good source of B vitamins, as well as being rich
in minerals. Wild rice is not in fact a rice but a grass and is high in
protein, making it lower GL than ordinary rice. It takes much longer
to cook, but look out for the quick-cook variety which is much
quicker than standard wild rice.

Serves 4
GL per serving: 10

175g wild rice (quick cook if possible), rinsed and drained
400g can aduki beans, rinsed and drained
4 tbsp pumpkin seeds
125g marinated artichoke hearts, drained and chopped
juice of 1 lemon
3 tbsp extra virgin olive oil, or to taste
rough handful of fresh flat-leaf parsley, finely chopped
salt and freshly ground black pepper

1. Cook the wild rice according to the pack instructions. Drain in
   a colander.
2. Stir the aduki beans into the rice and add the pumpkin seeds and
   artichoke hearts.
3. Squeeze in the lemon juice and add plenty of olive oil. Season to
   taste, sprinkle with parsley and serve.

Tip
Can be made in advance and served cold.

Butternut Squash and Tenderstem Broccoli Salad

The bright colours of the squash and broccoli in this salad are a good clue to its high antioxidant content. This can be served while the squash is still warm or at room temperature.

Serves 3–4
GL per serving (when serving 3): 3

½ butternut squash, unpeeled (see Tip), deseeded and cut into fairly thin slices
2 tsp dried oregano
2 tbsp light olive oil or virgin rapeseed oil
200g Tenderstem broccoli
about 115g mixed leaves, such as rocket, watercress, baby spinach and lamb's lettuce
2 tbsp roughly chopped sun-dried or sun-blush tomato pieces in oil, drained
50g walnut halves, roughly chopped
Vinaigrette (page 243), to serve

1. Preheat the oven to 220°C/425°F/Gas 7. Put the squash in a large bowl and toss with the oregano and oil to coat, then put on a baking tray. Roast for 25–30 minutes until tender, then set aside.
2. Steam the broccoli for 3 minutes or until just tender, then rinse in cold water to stop it cooking, and dry in a tea towel. Slice into sticks.
3. Put the leaves in a salad bowl, then add the squash and broccoli. Throw in the tomato and walnut pieces, then dress with the vinaigrette.

Tip
There is no need to peel the butternut squash unless you prefer to.

Peruvian Quinoa Salad

Quinoa is a healthier choice than bulgur wheat or couscous, as it is very high in protein, as well as containing minerals such as calcium and zinc. Pumpkin seeds further increase the mineral content of this recipe. Serve with green leaves or on its own.

Serves 4
GL per serving: 8

300g quinoa, rinsed
1 good handful of fresh coriander leaves, finely chopped
2 good handfuls of fresh flat-leaf parsley leaves, finely chopped
8 spring onions, finely sliced
1 garlic clove, crushed
4 tbsp pumpkin seeds
½ cucumber, finely diced
200g cherry tomatoes, thinly sliced or diced
juice of up to 4 limes, or to taste
2 ripe avocados, diced
good drizzle (about 4 tbsp) virgin rapeseed or olive oil
salt and freshly ground black pepper
Vinaigrette (page 243), to serve (optional)

1. Put the quinoa in a large saucepan, cover with double the amount of water and bring to the boil. Reduce the heat and simmer, covered, for 12–15 minutes until the water is absorbed and the grains are soft and fluffy.
2. Stir the fresh herbs through the quinoa along with the remaining ingredients, except the avocado and oil. Season to taste. When ready to serve, add the avocado and drizzle over the oil. Serve with vinaigrette, if you like.

Super-greens Salad

Sprouted beans are a very rich source of nutrients such as B vitamins, and the sprouting process makes the beans more digestible. This salad contains as many nutrient-dense ingredients as possible, making it a colourful blend of vitamins, fibre and antioxidants. Serve on a bed of dressed mixed leaves such as spinach, watercress, lamb's lettuce or rocket.

Serves 2
GL per serving: 2

1 tbsp light olive oil or virgin rapeseed oil
½ red onion, diced
115g mixed sprouts (such as sprouted aduki beans, chickpeas and lentils), rinsed and drained
1 tbsp walnuts, chopped
6 marinated sun-dried tomatoes, drained and finely chopped
1 tbsp pine nuts
1 tbsp extra virgin olive oil
1 tbsp finely chopped fresh flat-leaf parsley leaves
1 tbsp finely chopped fresh basil leaves
2 tsp dried oregano
2 tbsp lemon juice
1 large ripe avocado, diced
salt and freshly ground black pepper

1. Heat the oil in a frying pan. Add the onion and mixed sprouts, and stir-fry for 5 minutes (the sprouts do need cooking).
2. Add the nuts and stir-fry for a further minute.
3. Remove from the heat and put into a mixing bowl. Stir in the remaining ingredients, adding the avocado at the end in order not to make it too mushy. Season to taste and serve immediately.

Pesto Mushrooms on Grilled Polenta

Pre-cooked blocks of polenta are available in most supermarkets and delis, and they make a very easy, instant base for a starter or light meal such as this take on a toasted bruschetta.

Serves 4
GL per serving: 14

500g block of pre-cooked polenta, sliced into 8
1 tbsp light olive oil
450g mushrooms, sliced
4–5 tbsp vegan basil pesto, to taste
freshly ground black pepper
a handful of fresh basil leaves, roughly torn, to garnish

1. Preheat the grill to medium-high and grill the polenta slices for 5–8 minutes, turning halfway through, until each side starts to crisp and turn golden. You might have to do this in batches.
2. Meanwhile, heat the oil in a frying pan over a medium heat and cook the mushrooms for 5 minutes or until tender.
3. Stir the pesto into the mushrooms and then spoon the mixture onto the grilled polenta slices. Sprinkle with black pepper and basil leaves before serving.

Roasted Sweet Potato, Avocado and Pumpkin Seed Salad

This wonderfully colourful dish can either be served as a generous side salad or as a main meal. The different colours offer a range of phytonutrients. The herbs in the dressing can be varied or you can use any dark green leaves such as watercress, rocket or spinach.

Serves 2
GL per serving: 8.5

1 sweet potato, unpeeled
1 tbsp light olive oil
2 good handfuls of rocket
2 good handfuls of baby leaf spinach
225g cherry tomatoes, halved
1 ripe avocado, sliced
1 tbsp pumpkin seeds, toasted if you prefer

Dressing:
a handful each of fresh flat-leaf parsley and basil, very finely chopped
2 tbsp extra virgin olive oil
zest of ½ lemon
1 tbsp lemon juice, or to taste
salt and freshly ground black pepper

1. Preheat the oven to 200°C/400°F/Gas 6. Cut the sweet potato into long, evenly sized wedges, put them on a roasting tin, drizzle with the oil and toss to coat. Roast for 35 minutes.
2. Meanwhile, put the dressing ingredients in a small bowl or a screw-top jar and mix well. Season to taste.
3. Put the rocket, spinach and tomatoes in a salad bowl and toss together, then put on two plates.
4. Put the avocado over the mixed leaves. Top with the sweet potato wedges, scatter with the pumpkin seeds, then spoon the dressing generously over the top. Serve.

Tip
You can make the dressing in advance, but don't slice the avocado or construct the salad until just before serving.

Noodle Salad

This simple but oh-so-delicious salad makes great use of store-cupboard and fridge staples. The noodles plus chickpeas makes it a complete protein. It also features sprouted seeds, which are packed with enzymes and antioxidants, for a real nutrient boost. You can sprout seeds at home or buy them from health food shops, or simply use cress.

Serves 2
GL per serving: 11

90g soba or brown rice noodles
400g can chickpeas, rinsed and drained
½ red onion, finely diced
½ large cucumber, cut into matchstick strips
2 ripe tomatoes, diced
2.5cm root ginger, peeled and grated
2 heaped tbsp sprouted seeds such as broccoli or alfalfa
2 good handfuls of baby leaf spinach or watercress, finely chopped
3 tbsp sesame seeds

Dressing:
juice of 1 lime or lemon
a good drizzle of tamari or soy sauce, to taste
a good drizzle of toasted sesame oil, to taste

1. Cook the noodles in boiling water for 4–5 minutes or until just tender, or according to the pack instructions. Drain in a colander and refresh in cold water, then put them in a mixing bowl.
2. Add the remaining salad ingredients and toss well to mix thoroughly. Put the dressing ingredients in a small bowl or a screw-top jar and mix together well. Toss into the salad according to taste. Serve.

Sun-Dried Tomato and Pine Nut Stuffed Peppers

These easy-to-prepare roasted peppers are bursting with Mediterranean flavours and make a delicious light lunch. Brown basmati rice has a very low glycemic load so it provides longer-lasting energy. Serve with dark green leaves such as rocket, spinach and watercress, or Little Gem lettuce leaves.

Serves 2
GL per serving: 9

100g brown basmati rice, rinsed
½ tbsp coconut oil or light olive oil
1 red onion, finely chopped
2 garlic cloves, crushed
150g mushrooms
1 tbsp pine nuts
6 large pieces sun-dried tomato, finely chopped
1 tsp Italian mixed dried herbs, herbes de Provence, or oregano
a handful of fresh basil leaves or baby leaf spinach, chopped
2 large red peppers, halved lengthways and deseeded
salt and freshly ground black pepper
a handful of fresh basil leaves

1. Put the rice in a saucepan and cover generously with water. Bring to the boil, then reduce the heat slightly and cook for 25 minutes until tender. Drain in a colander.
2. Preheat the oven to 200°C/400°F/Gas 6. Heat the oil in a frying pan and gently cook the onion and garlic for 2 minutes. Add the mushrooms and fry for a further 3–5 minutes until softened.
3. Tip into a large bowl, and add the cooked rice, pine nuts, sun-dried tomatoes, dried herbs and basil. Season with salt and pepper to taste.
4. Stuff the peppers with the mixture, pressing it down to squash as

much in as possible. If you are preparing them in advance, store in the fridge until ready to cook (or you can also cook them in advance and serve them at room temperature).

5. Put on a baking tray and bake for 25–35 minutes or until the peppers look fairly soft. Serve sprinkled with the basil leaves.

Soups

Thai Mushroom Broth

Broths are fresh tasting and nutrient-rich because they are cooked so fast. This savoury Thai version contains mixed mushrooms such as shiitake, which have a smoky flavour and a high nutrient value.

Serves 2
GL per serving: 4

2 tsp vegetable bouillon powder
1 tsp mirin (Japanese rice cooking wine)
2 tsp tamari or soy sauce
1 garlic clove, finely sliced
1cm root ginger, peeled and finely sliced
50g mixed mushrooms (such as shiitake, oyster, chestnut),
    sliced or torn
4 pieces baby corn, chopped into thirds
1 tbsp chopped fresh coriander leaves
4 spring onions, sliced on the diagonal

1. Put all the ingredients, except the coriander and spring onions, in a small pan and add 300ml water. Bring to the boil, then reduce the heat and simmer, covered, for 5 minutes.
2. Add the coriander and spring onions, then stir and serve.

Avocado Gazpacho

Chilled soups are quick to make, nutrient-rich and ideal for entertaining, as they are easy to prepare in advance. Serve this deliciously fresh-tasting gazpacho straight from the fridge on a hot day.

Serves 2
GL per serving: 6

½ small red onion, chopped
½ red pepper, deseeded and chopped
I celery stick, sliced
5cm chunk of cucumber, quartered lengthways then finely sliced
    horizontally into small triangles
a good handful of cherry tomatoes
½ garlic clove, crushed
2 tsp deseeded and finely chopped mild red chilli
300ml tomato juice
juice of I lime
I tbsp finely chopped fresh coriander
I ripe avocado, peeled and chopped
freshly ground black pepper

1. Put all the ingredients, except the avocado and black pepper, in a bowl and stir together.
2. Using a blender or food processor, pulse the mixture to roughly blend it, but leave it fairly chunky for a good texture.
3. Stir in the avocado, sprinkle over the pepper and chill the soup in the fridge until ready to serve.

Leek and Potato Soup

This thick, satisfying soup, containing cannellini beans, is a complete, balanced meal.

Serves 2
GL per serving: 11

1 tsp coconut oil or light olive oil
2 garlic cloves, crushed
2 large leeks (300g trimmed weight), sliced
2 medium baby new potatoes, unpeeled and cubed
3 tsp vegetable bouillon powder
400g can cannellini beans, rinsed and drained
freshly ground black pepper

1. Heat the oil in a saucepan over a medium heat, add the garlic and cook for 30 seconds. Add the leeks, then cover and cook for 3 minutes or until softened.
2. Add the potatoes and 600ml boiling water to the pan, then stir in the bouillon powder. Bring to the boil, reduce the heat and simmer, covered, for 15 minutes.
3. Add the beans. Using a blender or food processor, whiz until fairly smooth. Season with pepper and serve.

Tip
Suitable for freezing.

Chestnut and Butter Bean Soup

Chestnuts have the lowest fat content of all nuts and a pleasantly sweet flavour that goes well with the smooth texture of the blended butter beans. This is fast, easy and deliciously filling.

Serves 4
GL per serving: 4

200g cooked and peeled chestnuts
400g can butter beans, rinsed and drained
1 onion, chopped
1 large carrot, chopped
3 tsp vegetable bouillon powder
freshly ground black pepper

1. Put all the ingredients, except for a handful of the chestnuts and the black pepper, in a saucepan. Add 600ml water, then bring to the boil. Reduce the heat and simmer, covered, for 15–20 minutes.
2. Using a blender or food processor, whiz until fairly smooth. Season with the black pepper, then sprinkle the reserved chestnuts on top. Serve.

Tip
Suitable for freezing.

Barley and Vegetable Broth

It's good to vary the grains you eat to make complete vegan proteins, and barley is a tasty one to try. This is a hearty, filling soup, and yet the GL is very low, thanks to the high vegetable content and the lentils and barley.

Serves 4
GL per serving: 5

2 tbsp light olive oil or coconut oil
2 carrots, diced
1 leek, thinly sliced

3 celery sticks, finely sliced
1 thyme sprig
115g pearl barley, rinsed and drained
50g red lentils, rinsed and drained
1.2 litres vegetable stock
2 tbsp finely chopped fresh flat-leaf parsley leaves
2 tbsp finely chopped baby spinach, watercress or rocket
salt and freshly ground black pepper

1. Heat the oil in a saucepan over a medium heat and cook the carrots, leek and celery for 5 minutes or until softened.
2. Stir in the thyme, barley, lentils and stock. Bring to the boil then reduce the heat and simmer, covered, for 45 minutes or until the pearl barley is soft to the bite and the vegetables are very tender.
3. Remove the thyme stalk, stir in the chopped parsley and greens, and season to taste. Serve.

Broccoli Soup

This is much better tasting than its simple ingredients would suggest, so do give it a try. It's a quick and easy way to increase your intake of greens. This recipe serves two because cooking it fresh each time gives you maximum benefit from the goodness of the broccoli.

Serves 2
GL per serving: 6

1 tbsp light olive oil, virgin rapeseed oil or coconut oil
2 garlic cloves, crushed
500ml vegetable stock
400g broccoli, cut into florets
100ml full-fat coconut milk or oat, rice or soya milk
salt and freshly ground black pepper

1. Heat the oil in a large saucepan over a medium heat, add the garlic and gently cook for 1 minute, taking care not to let it burn.
2. Add the stock and the broccoli. Bring it to the boil, then reduce the heat and simmer, covered, for 10 minutes or until the broccoli is tender.
3. Add the milk and plenty of black pepper, then whiz in a blender or food processor until smooth. Adjust the seasoning and serve.

Celeriac and Watercress Soup

A vegetable soup makes a tasty and sustaining vegan lunch, especially when made with vegetables such as celeriac, which has a good celery flavour and creates a rich and creamy soup.

Serves 3–4
GL per serving (when serving 3): 7

25g dairy-free spread or coconut oil
½ tbsp olive or virgin rapeseed oil
2 leeks, sliced
½ medium celeriac, peeled and diced
750ml vegetable stock
115g watercress
salt and freshly ground black pepper

1. Melt the dairy-free spread with the olive oil in a large saucepan over a medium heat, then add the leeks. Cover and cook for 10 minutes until softened.
2. Add the celeriac and stock. Bring to the boil, then reduce the heat and simmer, covered, for 15 minutes or until softened.
3. Add the watercress and blend until smooth. Season to taste and serve.

Tip
You can make this ahead. Blend after step 2, then freeze or chill.
Before serving, add the watercress, then blend again to maximise
the soup's goodness and colour.
  Suitable for freezing.

Beetroot and Borlotti Bean Soup

Bright purple, thick and filling, this soup can be served warm or
cold. You could save time by using cooked beetroot (without
vinegar), and blend it as soon as the onions have cooked. Borlotti
beans have a good, almost smoky, flavour and are a source of
B vitamins.

Serves 4
GL per serving: 6

1 tbsp light olive oil or virgin rapeseed oil
1 large or 2 small red onions, roughly chopped
2 garlic cloves, crushed
700g raw beetroot, peeled and diced
400g can borlotti beans, rinsed and drained
800ml vegetable stock
a large handful of fresh flat-leaf parsley, stalks removed
a large handful of fresh mint leaves
juice of 1 lemon
salt and freshly ground black pepper
4 tbsp soya or coconut yoghurt, to serve (optional)

1. Heat the oil in a large saucepan over a medium heat and cook
   the onion and garlic for 3–4 minutes until softened.
2. Add the beetroot, beans and stock. Bring to the boil, then reduce
   the heat and simmer, covered, for 15–20 minutes until the
   beetroot is fairly tender.

3. Add the herbs and lemon juice, then whiz in a blender or food processor until smooth.
4. Season to taste. Pour into bowls and add a dollop of yoghurt in the middle of each, if you like. Serve.

Tip
Suitable for freezing.

Chickpea, Carrot and Coriander Soup

This simple soup is quick and easy to make. Grating the carrots means that they soften very quickly – reducing the cooking time and therefore any loss of nutrients. Serve this soup on its own or with some crusty wholemeal bread or sourdough.

Serves 4
GL per serving: 6

400g can chickpeas, drained and rinsed
1 tbsp coconut oil or light olive oil
1 onion, finely sliced
4 carrots, coarsely grated
800ml vegetable stock
80g fresh coriander or fresh flat-leaf parsley, or a mixture
    of the two
1 tbsp extra virgin olive oil
2 tbsp lemon juice
salt and freshly ground black pepper

1. Put the chickpeas into a blender or food processor and whiz until smooth. If necessary, add a splash of water to get a puréed consistency.
2. Heat the oil in a large saucepan over a medium heat and cook the onion for 5 minutes or until softened.

3. Stir in the carrots then pour in the vegetable stock. Bring to the boil, then reduce the heat and simmer, covered, for 5 minutes. Stir in the puréed chickpeas and return to a simmer. Cook for a further 5 minutes or until the carrot tastes soft and a little sweet rather than coarse and raw. Season to taste.
4. Meanwhile, put the herbs, oil and lemon juice in a blender or food processor and blitz until the herbs are finely chopped and fairly smooth.
5. Ladle the soup into bowls and put a dollop of the herb garnish in the middle before sprinkling with a little black pepper. Serve.

Tip
The soup, but not the herb garnish, is suitable for freezing.

Spicy Gazpacho

This version of gazpacho contains a mixture of raw vegetables for extra flavour and nutrients. The base is, of course, tomatoes, which provide plenty of lycopene, the antioxidant known to mop up free radicals. It is traditionally served chilled, so you could pop it in the fridge for 30 minutes to an hour before serving, but it is also perfectly delicious eaten straight after it is made.

Serves 4
GL per serving: 6

3 red, yellow or orange peppers or a mixture of colours, deseeded and roughly chopped
1 cucumber, roughly chopped
1 red onion, roughly chopped
3 celery sticks, roughly chopped
400g ripe tomatoes
2 garlic cloves, crushed
2 long, mild red chillies, deseeded

125g Peppadew sweet baby peppers, drained weight, or hot pepper
   or chilli sauce to taste
2 handfuls of fresh coriander leaves
2 handfuls of fresh flat-leaf parsley leaves
2 ripe avocados, diced
400ml tomato juice
juice of 2 lemons
salt and freshly ground black pepper

1. Put the peppers in a food processor and add the cucumber,
   onion, celery, tomatoes, garlic, chillies, Peppadew peppers,
   coriander and parsley. Process to chop finely.
2. Add the avocados to the soup mixture, along with the tomato
   juice and lemon juice. Season to taste with salt and pepper, stir
   and serve.

Tip

If you prefer a milder flavour, don't add the Peppadew peppers or
hot pepper sauce but double the amount of avocado.
   Can be made in advance and chilled.

Spiced Butternut Squash Soup

This mildly spiced soup has a natural sweetness from the roasted
squash, and a rich, creamy texture from the coconut milk. Don't
buy reduced-fat coconut milk as coconut fat contains a beneficial fat
called lauric acid, which is antiviral and antibacterial.

Serves 4
GL per serving: 11

1kg butternut squash, unpeeled and cubed
2 tbsp, plus 2 tsp, light olive oil
1 tbsp curry powder (as hot as you prefer)

2 leeks, sliced
300ml vegetable stock, plus extra if needed
400ml can full-fat coconut milk
salt and freshly ground black pepper

1. Preheat the oven to 200°C/400°F/Gas 6. Put the squash in a
   bowl, sprinkle over 2 tablespoons of oil and the curry powder,
   and toss to coat. Spread the cubes over a baking tray or
   roasting tin and roast for 50 minutes, turning halfway through.
2. When the squash is cooked, put the leeks and the 2 teaspoons
   of oil in a large saucepan over a medium heat, and cook for 1
   minute, then cover and cook for 4 minutes or until softened.
3. Add the stock and coconut milk to the pan. Add the roasted
   butternut squash. Using a blender or food processor, whiz until
   smooth or your preferred consistency – you can add more stock
   to thin the soup if you prefer. Season to taste then bring up to
   temperature before serving, if necessary.

Tip
Suitable for freezing.

Lentil and Carrot Soup

This filling soup is mildly spiced with the warming flavours of cumin
and coriander and has a high fibre content. It's very quick and easy
to make. You could also throw in a handful of chopped parsley
and coriander if you like, before serving with chunks of your
favourite bread.

Serves 4
GL per serving: 6

2 tbsp light olive oil
2 garlic cloves, crushed

2 red onions, diced
2 tsp ground cumin
4 tsp ground coriander
200g red lentils, rinsed and drained
6 carrots, finely sliced
1.1 litre vegetable stock
salt and freshly ground black pepper

1. Heat the oil in a saucepan over a medium heat and cook the garlic and onions with the cumin and coriander for 5 minutes or until the onions are softened.
2. Add the lentils and carrots to the pan and pour in the stock. Bring to the boil, then reduce the heat and simmer, covered, for 20–30 minutes until the lentils have completely softened, stirring occasionally to prevent the soup from sticking.
3. Using a blender or food processor, whiz until smooth, then season to taste and serve.

Tip
Suitable for freezing.

Main meals

Pasta with Kale and Almonds

This dish is great for a warming winter supper and you can adapt the recipe according to taste or dietary requirements – use your preferred vegan pasta. The almonds add protein to the dish.

Serves 4
GL per serving: 10

400g of your choice of pasta such as wholewheat, brown rice pasta
   or buckwheat pasta (fusilli or penne both work well)
extra virgin olive oil, to drizzle
125g kale, washed and tough stems removed, chopped
75g flaked almonds
2 tsp vegetable bouillon powder
2 tbsp tahini
salt and freshly ground black pepper

1. Preheat the oven to 200°C/400°F/Gas 6. Cook the pasta in
   boiling salted water according to the pack instructions. Drain
   in a colander, then return it to the pan and drizzle with a little
   extra virgin olive oil. Grind over some black pepper then cover
   with a lid.
2. Meanwhile, put the kale in a roasting tin, drizzle with oil, then
   season generously with salt. Roast for 5 minutes or until it is
   starting to just dry out and crisp up.
3. Lightly toast the almonds in a dry frying pan over a medium heat
   for 2 minutes or until just starting to turn golden.
4. Put the bouillon powder and tahini in a small bowl and add
   2 tablespoons hot water. Stir to make a creamy, fairly smooth
   sauce. Taste and adjust the seasoning and consistency as
   necessary (some tahini is stronger than others, so you might
   prefer a little more water or more bouillon powder).
5. Toss the flaked almonds and kale through the pasta and stir in the
   tahini sauce, then serve.

Beetroot and Celeriac Roast

This is a satisfying supper or weekend roast on its own for two
or you can serve it for more people as an accompaniment. Any
leftovers can easily be reheated. Celeriac and beetroot are healthy
low-carb starchy vegetables and the dish has a little added protein
from the walnuts.

Serves 2
GL per serving: 7

½ celeriac, peeled and cut into bite-sized pieces
2 raw beetroot, topped but unpeeled, cut into bite-sized pieces
2 red onions, cut into bite-sized pieces
2 garlic cloves, sliced
a good drizzle of extra virgin olive oil
½ Savoy cabbage, outer leaves, heart and any thick stems removed,
    sliced fairly thinly
50g walnut halves
salt and freshly ground black pepper

1. Preheat the oven to 200°C/400°F/Gas 6. Put the celeriac,
   beetroot and onions in a roasting tin and add the garlic, then
   drizzle generously with oil. Stir and season with salt.
2. Roast for 20 minutes or until the root vegetables feel fairly soft
   when pierced with a knife.
3. Add the cabbage leaves and a little more oil and salt, then stir
   loosely to combine and coat. Return to the oven for 10 minutes
   or until the cabbage is starting to look cooked and toasted at
   the edges.
4. Scatter the walnuts over the dish, stir again to combine and
   return to the oven for a further 5 minutes or until the nuts
   are toasted.
5. Remove from the oven, sprinkle with black pepper, then taste
   and adjust the seasoning. Serve.

Sun-Blush Tomato and Black Olive Chickpea Salad

This strongly flavoured salad combines Middle Eastern and
Mediterranean flavours very successfully. Serve with sourdough
bread or oatcakes.

Serves 2
GL per serving: 8

400g can chickpeas, rinsed and drained
2 tsp sun-blush tomatoes in oil (reserve the oil as a
    dressing), chopped
2 tsp dry pitted black olives (packed without oil or brine), chopped
4 spring onions, finely sliced on the diagonal
1 tsp finely chopped fresh flat-leaf parsley leaves
2 tsp lemon juice
2 tsp tahini
2 tsp oil from the jar of sun-blush tomatoes or extra virgin olive oil
freshly ground black pepper

Put all the ingredients into a large bowl and mix well together.
Season with black pepper. Chill lightly or serve immediately.

Roasted Chickpea and Lemon Tabbouleh

When roasted, chickpeas develop a lovely chewy yet crunchy
texture. Enlivened with lemon and spices, they are delicious in this
tabbouleh salad.

Serves 2
GL per serving: 10

140g quinoa, rinsed
1 tsp vegetable bouillon powder
400g can chickpeas, rinsed and drained
2 tbsp light olive oil
1 tsp ground cumin
1 garlic clove, crushed
zest of ½ a lemon and juice of 1 lemon
1 tbsp sesame seeds

2 tbsp chopped fresh flat-leaf parsley leaves
freshly ground black pepper

1. Preheat the oven to 200°C/400°F/Gas 6. Put the quinoa and bouillon powder in a large saucepan, cover with double the amount of water and bring to the boil. Reduce the heat and simmer, covered, for 12–15 minutes until the water is absorbed and the grains are soft and fluffy.
2. Meanwhile, put the chickpeas in a bowl and toss them in 1 tablespoon of the oil, with the cumin, garlic, lemon zest and juice, and sesame seeds.
3. Tip the chickpeas into a roasting tin and roast for 30 minutes, shaking halfway through (the sesame seeds should turn golden but not burn).
4. Mix the chickpeas into the cooked quinoa with the parsley. Season with black pepper and stir in the remaining 1 tablespoon of oil. Serve.

Vegetable Chilli

Packed with beans, vegetables and spices, this is a hearty chilli. It's even better served with quinoa to make it protein rich.

Serves 4
GL per serving: 6

2 tsp coconut oil or light olive oil
1 onion, chopped
2 garlic cloves, crushed
1 red pepper, deseeded and chopped
1 tsp ground cumin
1 tsp crushed chilli flakes
1 tsp chilli powder
250g mushrooms, sliced

400g can chopped tomatoes
3 tbsp tomato purée
400g can kidney beans, rinsed and drained
400g can borlotti beans, rinsed and drained
3 tsp vegetable bouillon powder
freshly ground black pepper

1. Heat the oil in a saucepan over a medium heat, add the onion and garlic and cook for 2 minutes.
2. Add the chopped pepper and spices, then cover and cook for 5 minutes or until the pepper softens.
3. Add the mushrooms and cook for 1 minute until they soften.
4. Tip in the chopped tomatoes, tomato purée, beans and bouillon powder. Season with pepper and stir. Bring to the boil, then reduce the heat and simmer, covered, for 5 minutes. Serve.

Bean-Stuffed Aubergines

A rich, tomatoey stuffing brings this baked aubergine to life. Bursting with antioxidants from the onions, garlic, mushrooms and tomatoes, this makes a lovely, simple supper for two.

Serves 2
GL per serving: 7

1 aubergine
2 tsp coconut oil or light olive oil, plus 1 tsp olive oil for brushing
2 garlic cloves, crushed
2 red onions, chopped
100g button mushrooms, sliced
1 red pepper, deseeded and chopped fairly small
200g tomato passata
½ × 400g can borlotti beans, rinsed and drained
1 tsp herbes de Provence

I tsp vegetable bouillon powder
salt and freshly ground black pepper

1. Preheat the oven to 190°C/375°F/Gas 5. Cut the aubergine
   in half and scoop out the flesh with a teaspoon to use in the
   stuffing, taking care not to puncture the skin. Put the shells
   to one side.
2. For the stuffing, heat the 2 teaspoons of oil in a saucepan over a
   medium heat, add the garlic and cook for 30 seconds, then add
   the onions and cook for 2 minutes.
3. Add the mushrooms, the reserved aubergine flesh and the red
   pepper, and cook for 10 minutes or until they soften slightly.
4. Add the tomato passata, beans, herbs and bouillon powder.
   Season with salt and pepper to taste and stir. Bring to the boil,
   then reduce the heat and simmer, covered, for 2 minutes.
5. Brush the outside of the reserved aubergine shells with the
   I tsp olive oil and put them in a roasting tin, then stuff the shells
   with the filling. (If you have any left over, it's delicious with baked
   potatoes or pasta.) Cover the roasting tin with kitchen foil and
   bake for 40–45 minutes, until the aubergine is tender. Serve.

Mediterranean Bean Feast

Beans are a great ingredient for vegan meals because they are
versatile and go well with so many flavours. A Mediterranean mix is
probably the most popular, as tomatoes, artichokes and olives make
such a rich combination. Served with a grain this makes a quick and
simple but nourishing meal.

Serves 2
GL per serving: 7

I tsp light olive oil
I red onion, chopped

400g can mixed pulses, drained and rinsed
2 tbsp good-quality tomato-based pasta sauce
4 marinated artichoke hearts from a jar
a handful of black olives, pitted and roughly chopped
a handful of fresh basil leaves, torn
freshly ground black pepper

1. Heat the oil in a saucepan over a medium heat, add the onion
   and gently cook for 1–2 minutes, just to take the raw edge off.
2. Add the mixed pulses, tomato sauce, artichoke hearts and olives,
   and stir. Season with pepper, then remove from the heat and add
   the basil leaves. Leave to rest for a little while, if possible, to allow
   the flavours to develop before serving.

Asparagus and Flageolet Bean Risotto

This gorgeous spring risotto is studded with green from the
asparagus tips, flageolet beans and herbs. The brown basmati rice,
which has the lowest GL score of all rice varieties, is just as creamy
as Arborio rice, the traditional risotto rice, thanks to the addition of
tahini white sauce. This meal is a complete vegan protein, nourishing
and full of flavour.

Serves 2
GL per serving: 10

100g brown basmati rice
2 tsp vegetable bouillon powder
100g asparagus tips
400g can flageolet beans, rinsed and drained
2 handfuls of rocket, torn
2 tsp lemon juice
1 tbsp chopped fresh flat-leaf parsley leaves or chives
freshly ground black pepper

Tahini white sauce:
2 tbsp cornflour
420ml soya milk or nut milk
2 tbsp tahini
4 tsp vegetable bouillon powder

1. Put the rice in a large saucepan and add the bouillon powder and 210ml water. Bring to the boil, then reduce the heat and simmer, covered, for 15–20 minutes until the water is absorbed and the rice is al dente – tender but retains a bite.
2. While the rice is cooking, steam the asparagus for 7–8 minutes, until tender but not collapsing.
3. Meanwhile, make the sauce. Put the cornflour in a small bowl and stir in half the milk. Mix until smooth. Pour into a saucepan and add the tahini and bouillon powder, then cook over a gentle heat for 3–5 minutes, stirring constantly and gradually adding the remaining milk to make a smooth, thick sauce.
4. Put the cooked rice in a bowl and mix in the flageolet beans, asparagus, rocket, lemon juice, herbs and hot sauce, stirring to allow the rocket to wilt slightly in the heat. Season with black pepper, then serve.

Cashew and Sesame Quinoa

The sesame oil, soy sauce and cashew nuts enliven this dish, while the raw veg provide extra crunch as well as vitamins and antioxidants. Nuts are a very useful food for vegans because they add protein and healthy fats, and are full of flavour.

Serves 2
GL per serving: 6

140g quinoa
1 tsp vegetable bouillon powder

4 tbsp fresh or frozen petits pois
2 tbsp cashew nuts
2 tsp sesame oil
1 tbsp tamari or soy sauce
2 tsp lemon juice
1 large carrot, cut into matchstick strips
6 spring onions, finely sliced on the diagonal
freshly ground black pepper

1. Put the quinoa and bouillon powder in a large saucepan
   and cover with double the amount of water. Bring to the
   boil, then reduce the heat and simmer, covered, for
   12–13 minutes until the water is absorbed and the grains are
   soft and fluffy.
2. Add the peas and stir through, then remove from the heat. They
   will cook or soften slightly in the residual warmth.
3. Combine with the remaining ingredients, tossing thoroughly to
   mix all the flavours and allow the quinoa to absorb the liquid
   seasonings. Serve.

Simple Lentil Dahl

This easy recipe is very moreish, low GL, and incredibly rich in
antioxidants. Lentils are one of the cheapest and easiest nourishing
vegan foods. To make this into a complete protein, serve with pitta
bread or a grain such as brown rice or quinoa.

Serves 4
GL per serving: 7

300g red lentils, rinsed and drained
1 onion, chopped
4 garlic cloves, crushed
4 tsp vegetable bouillon powder

400g can chopped tomatoes
1 heaped tsp curry powder

1. Put the lentils in a saucepan and add 600ml water, the onion, garlic and bouillon powder. Bring to the boil, then reduce the heat and simmer, covered, for 10 minutes.
2. Add the tomatoes and curry powder, and stir well. Cover and leave to simmer for a further 20 minutes, stirring occasionally to make sure it doesn't stick to the bottom of the pan. If it starts to get too thick, add a little water; if it seems too watery, leave uncovered. The lentils should form a porridge-like consistency. Serve.

Cauliflower Dhal

The addition of ginger and turmeric provides a spicy edge to this variation on the traditional dhal theme. The al dente cauliflower – a super-healthy cruciferous vegetable rich in vitamins and containing protein – provides bite and contrasts deliciously with the smooth lentils.

Serves 2
GL per serving: 3

2 onions, chopped
2 garlic cloves, crushed
2cm root ginger, peeled and grated
½ tsp turmeric
½ tsp ground cumin
¼ tsp cayenne pepper
2 tsp coconut oil or olive oil
75g red lentils, rinsed and drained
2 tsp vegetable bouillon powder
⅓ medium-sized cauliflower, cut into small florets

1. Put the onions into a blender or food processor and add the garlic, ginger, turmeric, cumin and cayenne pepper. Whiz to a purée.
2. Heat the oil in a saucepan over a medium heat and add the onion mixture. Cook for 5 minutes, then add the lentils, 600ml water and the bouillon powder. Bring to the boil, then reduce the heat and simmer, uncovered, for 10 minutes.
3. Add the cauliflower, and return it to the boil, then reduce the heat and simmer, covered, for 15 minutes, to allow the lentils to cook down to almost a purée and for the cauliflower to soften. Serve.

Tip
Suitable for freezing.

Lentil Stew

This thick, rich stew is ideal for cold nights. Red lentils are very low GL so they make a healthy vegan choice – and are useful if you are trying to lose weight. This recipe serves four, but if you're serving fewer people you can have it again the next day or freeze the remainder.

Serves 4
GL per serving: 5

1 tsp coconut oil or olive oil
1 garlic clove, crushed
1 onion, chopped
1 green pepper, deseeded and chopped
1 small carrot, sliced
1 celery stick, sliced
125g red lentils, rinsed and drained
2½ tsp vegetable bouillon powder

1 tsp dried mixed Italian herbs
12 cherry tomatoes, roughly chopped
1½ tbsp tomato purée
freshly ground black pepper

1. Heat the oil in a large frying pan over a medium heat and add the garlic. Cook for 30 seconds or so, then add the onion and cook gently for 2 minutes.
2. Add the green pepper, carrot and celery, and cook for a further 5 minutes.
3. Add the lentils, bouillon powder, 180ml water and the herbs to the pan, and stir well. Bring to the boil, then cook, uncovered, for 10 minutes.
4. Add the tomatoes and tomato purée to the pan, then reduce the heat and simmer, covered, for a further 15–20 minutes until the stew is thick and the lentils are completely soft. Season with black pepper and serve.

Teriyaki Tofu

In this simple dish the fabulous flavour of Japanese teriyaki sauce transforms plain tofu, which readily takes on other flavours. Tofu, a complete protein, is a good mainstay food in a vegan diet. Serve with stir-fried or steam-fried vegetables (see page 239).

Serves 2
GL per serving: 4

250g pack plain organic tofu, patted dry with kitchen
   towel and cubed
1 tbsp coconut oil or olive oil

Teriyaki sauce:
2 tbsp tamari or soy sauce

2 tbsp mirin (Japanese rice cooking wine)
2.5cm root ginger, peeled and grated
1 tsp xylitol

1. Put the ingredients for the sauce in a small bowl and mix well. Put the tofu in a shallow dish and add the teriyaki sauce. Leave to marinate in the fridge for 30 minutes.
2. Heat the oil in a large frying pan over a medium heat. Using a slotted spoon, take the tofu out of the marinade, reserving this for later. Stir-fry the tofu on all sides.
3. When the tofu starts to turn a pale golden colour, remove it from the heat and pour the reserved marinade into the pan. Return to the heat for a few seconds to thicken, then serve.

Marinated Tofu Couscous

Here is a ridiculously easy meal – the couscous cooks in 4 minutes and the tofu pieces are simply stirred in. Lemon, herbs and fresh veg add extra flavour and bite. This dish is ideal for an impromptu al fresco lunch or to take to work.

Serves 2
GL per serving: 12

100g Belazu barley couscous (or regular wheat couscous)
1½ tsp vegetable bouillon powder
150g pack marinated tofu, cubed
2 tsp lemon juice
5 spring onions, finely chopped on the diagonal
6 cherry tomatoes, thinly sliced
½ tbsp fresh flat-leaf parsley leaves finely chopped

1. Cook the couscous by placing it in a bowl and adding boiling water to just cover it. Add the bouillon powder, stir, then cover

with a clean tea towel for 4 minutes to allow it to soften and absorb the water.

2. When the couscous is ready, stir it through with a fork to break up the grains, then mix in the remaining ingredients and serve.

Vegetable Steam-fry

Serve this vegetable-rich steam-fry with quinoa to boost the protein content. Vary the vegetables according to taste but try to include a range of different colours so that you benefit from the full spectrum of antioxidants.

Serves 2
GL per serving: 4

1 tbsp virgin rapeseed oil or coconut oil
2 garlic cloves, finely sliced
½ red chilli, or to taste, deseeded and finely chopped
1 bunch of spring onions, finely sliced
75g cashew nuts
1 tbsp tamari or soy sauce
1 tbsp mirin (Japanese rice cooking wine)
1 tbsp rice vinegar
1 carrot, cut into matchstick strips
2 heads of pak choi, sliced
200g beansprouts
100ml vegetable stock, if needed

1. Heat the oil in a hot wok over a medium heat, swirl it about to coat the base and sides, then throw in the garlic, chilli, spring onions and cashew nuts, and stir-fry for 10 seconds. Add the soy sauce, mirin and rice vinegar.

2. Add the carrot, pak choi and beansprouts, and cover with a lid (or 2 sheets of kitchen paper doused in water if your wok does

not have a lid) to let the vegetables steam-fry for 2 minutes or until al dente, adding the stock to keep it moist if necessary.
3. Remove the kitchen paper, stir and serve.

Lentil and Sweet Potato Dahl

There are countless recipes for this Indian staple, which is traditionally served as a milder accompaniment to curries, but if you add plenty of spices, garlic and ginger it is very good served on its own with rice and perhaps some finely diced red onion, tomato and cucumber.

Serves 4
GL per serving: 6

1 tbsp virgin rapeseed oil or coconut oil
1 tsp ground turmeric
1 tsp ground cumin
2 tsp garam masala
1 garlic clove, crushed
1 red onion, diced
2cm root ginger, peeled and grated
1 carrot, thinly sliced
165g red lentils, rinsed and drained
750ml vegetable stock
1 sweet potato, cubed into small pieces (see Tip)
2 handfuls of baby spinach, shredded
juice of ½ lemon
salt and freshly ground black pepper

1. Heat the oil in a large frying pan over a medium heat. Add the spices, garlic, onion and ginger, and fry for 1 minute. Add the carrot and lentils, stir and pour in the stock.
2. Bring to the boil, boil rapidly for 10 minutes, then reduce

the heat to a simmer. Add the sweet potato, stir, and cook for a further 15 minutes or until the lentils and sweet potato are soft.

3. Stir in the spinach and let it wilt, then add the lemon juice and season to taste before serving.

Tip
Peel the sweet potato if you prefer the look and texture of it, otherwise leave it unpeeled.

Suitable for freezing.

Bean and Mushroom Bolognese

This thick, hearty bean stew works well with pasta and a rocket, watercress and spinach salad. The beans and mushrooms make it high in B vitamins. If you cannot get hold of pinto beans, borlotti beans are also delicious.

Serves 4
GL per serving: 7

2 tbsp light olive oil, virgin rapeseed oil or coconut oil
1 large red onion, diced
2 garlic cloves, crushed
350g mushrooms, thinly sliced
350g tomato passata
400g can pinto beans, rinsed and drained
2 tsp vegetable bouillon powder
2 tsp dried oregano
freshly ground black pepper

1. Heat the oil in a large saucepan over a medium heat, and cook the onion and garlic for 10 or minutes until softened. Add the mushrooms and cook for 5 minutes.

2. Add the passata, beans, bouillon and oregano, and bring to the
   boil, then reduce the heat and simmer, covered, for 20 minutes
   or until the sauce has reduced slightly and the vegetables are soft.
   Season to taste and serve.

Tip
Suitable for freezing.

Sweet Potato and Chickpea Stew

You can also use pumpkin or squash instead of sweet potato for this
warming stew, if you prefer. Serve with a mixture of brown basmati
rice and wild rice, and a green salad.

Serves 4
GL per serving: 8

1 tbsp light olive oil, virgin rapeseed oil or coconut oil
1 red onion, finely sliced
1 garlic clove, crushed
1cm root ginger, peeled and grated
½ red chilli, deseeded and finely chopped
1 tsp ground turmeric
½ tsp smoked paprika
1 large sweet potato, unpeeled, diced
1 red pepper, deseeded and cut into small dice
400g can chickpeas, rinsed and drained
400g can chopped tomatoes
150ml vegetable stock
freshly ground black pepper
salt
squeeze of lemon juice, to serve

1. Heat the oil in a large saucepan over a medium heat and cook the onion for 10 minutes or until softened.
2. Add the garlic, ginger, chilli, turmeric and smoked paprika, and stir for 1 minute.
3. Add the sweet potato and red pepper, and cook for a further 5 minutes to let the vegetables start to colour.
4. Add the chickpeas, tomatoes and stock. Bring to the boil, then reduce the heat and simmer, covered, for 20 minutes or until the sweet potato is tender.
5. Season to taste and squeeze some fresh lemon juice over the top before serving.

Tip
Suitable for freezing.

Quinoa Pilaf with Red Pepper and Pumpkin Seeds

The protein food, quinoa, is also a good source of valuable minerals such as calcium and zinc. Combining it with pumpkin seeds makes this dish even richer in protein.

Serves 4
GL per serving: 5

1 tbsp light olive oil, virgin rapeseed oil or coconut oil
1 red onion, finely diced
1 red pepper, deseeded and finely diced
175g quinoa, rinsed and drained
450ml vegetable stock
40g pumpkin seeds
a good handful of finely chopped fresh flat-leaf parsley leaves
a good handful of finely chopped baby spinach
a squeeze of lemon juice
salt and freshly ground black pepper

1. Heat the oil in a large saucepan or frying pan with a lid over a medium heat, add the onion and pepper and cook for 10 minutes or until softened.
2. Add the quinoa and stock. Bring to the boil, then reduce the heat and simmer, covered, for 12–15 minutes or until the quinoa has absorbed the water and softened.
3. Stir in the pumpkin seeds, parsley and spinach, then season to taste and add a squeeze of lemon juice. Serve.

Sun-Dried Tomato Pesto with Cannellini Beans

This easy and delicious pesto is great stirred through pasta, quinoa or, as in this recipe, mixed with beans. You won't need all the pesto for this recipe, so try leftovers dolloped onto a baked sweet potato with salad or simply spread on bread – delicious!

Serves 2 (with leftover pesto)
GL per serving: 8

50g toasted pine nuts
20 large sun-dried tomatoes
4 tbsp cider vinegar
1 tbsp Dijon mustard
6 garlic cloves, crushed
300ml extra virgin olive or virgin rapeseed oil, or ideally a
    blend of both
400g can cannellini beans, rinsed and drained
salt and freshly ground black pepper

1. Lightly toast the pine nuts in a dry frying pan over a medium heat until golden – watch carefully to stop them scorching.
2. Put the tomatoes in a food processor or blender and add the vinegar, mustard and garlic. Whiz to form a paste, then season to taste with salt and pepper.

3. Pour in the oil and slowly blend until fairly smooth. Taste and adjust the seasoning if necessary.
4. Put the beans in a bowl, then stir about a quarter (about 6 tablespoons or to taste) of the pesto into the beans and crush with a potato masher. (Alternatively, lightly blitz in the food processor.) Keep the remaining pesto in an airtight container in the fridge for easy meals.

Tip
The pesto keeps for ten days in an airtight container in the fridge. Suitable for freezing.

Tofu Noodle Stir-fry

The protein-rich tofu in this recipe is packed with flavour from the ginger, garlic, soy and sesame.

Serves 2
GL per serving: 10

400g firm tofu, patted dry with kitchen paper and cut into bite-sized cubes
2 tbsp sesame seeds
150g soba noodles
4 tbsp coconut oil or virgin rapeseed oil
1cm root ginger, peeled and grated
1 red onion, sliced
1 carrot, finely sliced
150g sugar snap peas
150g beansprouts, rinsed
2 tbsp tamari or soy sauce
2 tbsp rice vinegar
200ml vegetable stock
juice of 1 lime

Marinade:

1 tbsp toasted sesame oil

2.5cm root ginger, peeled and grated

2 garlic cloves, crushed

2 tbsp tamari or soy sauce

2 tsp rice wine vinegar

1 tsp chilli-infused oil

1. To make the marinade, put all the ingredients in a shallow bowl and mix together. Stir in the tofu to coat thoroughly, then put it in the fridge for at least 1 hour and preferably 3 hours or more.
2. Meanwhile, put the sesame seeds in a small pan over a medium heat and toast them lightly for 1 minute, shaking the pan frequently. Leave to one side.
3. Cook the noodles in boiling water for 4–5 minutes or until just tender, or according to the pack instructions, drain in a colander and leave to one side.
4. Drain the tofu when ready to use, reserving the drained marinade for later. Heat 2 tablespoons of oil in a wok over a medium-high heat, add the tofu and stir-fry for 3 minutes, stirring gently, as the tofu will be very soft. Remove from the wok and leave to one side on a plate.
5. Heat the remaining 2 tablespoons of oil in the wok, add the ginger and onion, and stir-fry for 1 minute. Add the carrot and stir-fry for another 2 minutes, then add the sugar snap peas. Stir-fry for a further 5 minutes before adding the cooked noodles and beansprouts to the wok. Stir-fry to reheat and combine.
6. Pour in the soy sauce, rice vinegar, stock and remaining marinade, then stir and simmer for 1 minute.
7. Ladle the stir-fry into two bowls and squeeze a little lime juice over. Sprinkle the toasted sesame seeds on top of each portion before serving.

Sesame Soba Noodle Salad

Nutty-flavoured soba noodles are made from buckwheat and are here combined with smoked tofu to make a protein-rich meal. The ginger and soy add richness to the flavour, and it's also rich in zinc. Accompany this with some stir-fried green vegetables for extra nutrients.

Serves 4
GL per serving: 9

400g soba noodles
4 tbsp sesame seeds
60g root ginger, peeled and grated
4 tbsp toasted sesame oil
4 tbsp freshly squeezed lime or lemon juice
4 tbsp tamari or soy sauce
400g firm smoked tofu, cubed
½ large cucumber, very finely sliced

1. Cook the noodles in boiling water for 4–5 minutes or until just tender, or according to the pack instructions. Drain in a colander, refresh in cold water, and transfer to a large bowl. Meanwhile, put the sesame seeds in a small pan over a medium heat and toast them lightly for 1 minute, shaking the pan frequently. Leave to one side.
2. To make the dressing, put the ginger in a blender and add the sesame oil, lime juice and soy sauce. Whiz until smooth. (Some bits of ginger will probably remain, which is fine.)
3. Pour the dressing over the noodles, add the tofu cubes and cucumber slices, then toss together. Serve in bowls and scatter with the toasted sesame seeds.

Baked Falafel

These are delicious with a dollop of coconut yoghurt and a salad of red onion, tomato and coriander, and either stuffed in a toasted wholemeal pitta or served with quinoa or couscous. Serve with a large wedge of lemon per person to squeeze over the top and bring out the flavour.

Serves 4
GL per serving: 6

2 tbsp ground flaxseed
2 × 400g cans chickpeas, rinsed and drained
4 garlic cloves, crushed
4 tsp tahini
10 spring onions, roughly chopped
50g sesame seeds, plus 60g sesame seeds for coating
4 tsp ground cumin
2 tsp ground coriander
2 tbsp finely chopped fresh flat-leaf parsley leaves
2 tsp salt
freshly ground black pepper

1. Put the flaxseed in a bowl and add 90ml of cold water. Leave to soak for 20 minutes to thicken. Set aside.
2. Preheat the oven to 200°C/400°F/Gas 6. Line a baking tray with baking paper.
3. Put the chickpeas in a food processor and add the garlic, tahini, spring onions, the 50g sesame seeds, spices and parsley. Whiz until fairly smooth and combined. Taste and season with salt and pepper.
4. Stir in the flaxseed mixture and shape into 16 balls, roughly the size of golf balls.
5. Put the 60g of sesame seeds onto a plate and roll the balls in them. This is a bit fiddly, so it might be necessary to then reshape the falafel in your hand.

6. Put the balls on the prepared baking tray and bake for
   20–25 minutes or until just golden on top and firm to the touch.

Tip
Suitable for freezing.

Quinoa with Sun-Blush Tomatoes and Olives

Lots of herbs and leaves, plus garlic, make this simple recipe a
great source of antioxidants, and the quinoa contains all the eight
essential amino acids that make up a complete protein. This is a
light dish, so try it with a mixed salad and avocado slices or perhaps
a corn on the cob or some toasted wholemeal pitta bread to make
it more filling.

Serves 4
GL per serving: 8

300g quinoa, rinsed
1 tbsp coconut oil or light olive oil
1 red onion, diced
2 courgettes, diced
juice of 1 lemon
2 handfuls of fresh basil leaves
2 handfuls of fresh flat-leaf parsley leaves
2 handfuls of rocket and/or watercress
2 handfuls of baby leaf spinach
1 garlic clove, crushed
175g pitted Kalamata olives
175g sun-blush tomatoes
freshly ground black pepper

1. Put the quinoa in a large saucepan, add double the amount
   of water and bring it to the boil. Cover and simmer for

12–15 minutes or until the water is absorbed and the grains are soft and fluffy.

2. Meanwhile, heat the oil in a large frying pan over a medium heat, add the onion and courgettes and cook for 1 minute, then cover and cook for 5 minutes or until softened.
3. Put the lemon juice in a blender or food processer and add the herbs and leaves, garlic and some black pepper, then blitz until the leaves are finely chopped. Add the olives and sun-blush tomatoes, and blend briefly until they are coarsely chopped and combined.
4. Stir the cooked vegetables and the olive mixture into the quinoa and taste to check the seasoning. Serve warm or cold.

Mushroom and Pot Barley Risotto

Barley doesn't need nearly as much attention during cooking as traditional risotto rice – just pour on the stock and wait for it to be absorbed. Pot barley is a good source of protein, fibre and niacin (vitamin B3). It needs soaking overnight or for at least six hours, but simply cover it with boiling water, leave it to soak and drain it the next day. This makes the barley more digestible and reduces the cooking time.

Serves 4
GL per serving: 7

300g pot barley
25g dried porcini mushrooms
vegetable stock as needed
2 tbsp coconut oil or light olive oil
2 onions, finely chopped
300g assorted fresh mushrooms, sliced
2 tbsp finely chopped fresh flat-leaf parsley leaves
salt and freshly ground black pepper

1. Start the night before. Put the pot barley in a large bowl, pour over hot water to cover generously and leave to soak overnight.

2. The next day, put the porcini in a bowl and add warm water to cover. Leave to soak for 30 minutes. Drain in a sieve and reserve the liquid. Drain the barley in a colander, reserving the liquid. Put the mushroom liquid and barley soaking liquid in a measuring jug and top up with stock to measure 1.2 litres. Pour into a saucepan. Bring to the boil, then reduce the heat to a simmer.

3. Heat the oil in a heavy-based saucepan over a medium heat, add the onions and cook for 4 minutes or until softened. Add the fresh mushrooms and cook for another 6–8 minutes until softened.

4. Pour in the pot barley and stir frequently for 2 minutes to toast the grains.

5. Add the porcini mushrooms and cook for 2 minutes, stirring occasionally. Add the stock and bring to the boil, then reduce the heat and simmer for 1 hour, stirring occasionally, until it has absorbed all the liquid.

6. Season to taste with salt and black pepper and serve scattered with the parsley.

Lentil and Squash Curry

This curry is very easy to make and is bursting with flavour from the spices, garlic, onion and spinach. It's also jam-packed with fibre to aid digestion, and vitamins and phytonutrients (plant nutrients). Serve with brown basmati rice for a protein-packed vegan main meal.

Serves 4
GL per serving: 10

1 tbsp light olive oil
2 red onions, chopped

4 garlic cloves, crushed
1 butternut squash, unpeeled, cubed
2 tbsp curry powder
600ml vegetable stock
100g dried red lentils, rinsed and drained
400g can tomatoes, chopped
a large handful of baby leaf spinach
2 tsp sea salt
a handful of fresh coriander, finely chopped
freshly ground black pepper

1. Heat the oil in a saucepan over a medium heat, add the onions
   and garlic and cook for 5 minutes or until softened.
2. Stir in the butternut squash and curry powder, then pour in
   the stock, lentils and tomatoes, and bring to the boil. Cover and
   simmer for 1 hour or until the squash is softened and the sauce
   reduced, stirring occasionally.
3. Stir in the spinach, cover for a few minutes while it wilts, then
   season to taste with the salt, pepper and coriander. Serve.

Tip
Suitable for freezing, but don't add the spinach until you've defrosted
and reheated the curry.

Chickpea and Cauliflower Curry

India has some of the finest vegan dishes in the world, packed with
flavour, thanks to the liberal use of herbs and spices combined with
vegetables. This curry is very quick to make. Serve it with brown
basmati rice or quinoa.

Serves 4
GL per serving: 7

2 tbsp coconut oil or light olive oil
3 tbsp medium curry paste
2 large onions, sliced
½ cauliflower, broken into small florets
400g can chickpeas, rinsed and drained
400ml can full-fat coconut milk
210ml vegetable stock
1 tbsp tamari or soy sauce
250g fine green beans
salt
handful of fresh coriander leaves, torn or roughly chopped,
    to garnish

1. Put the oil and the curry paste in a large frying pan or wok over
   a medium heat, add the onions and fry for 5 minutes or until
   softened. Add the cauliflower and chickpeas to the pan and stir
   to coat them in the other ingredients.
2. Pour in the coconut milk, stock and soy sauce, and stir. Bring
   to the boil, then reduce the heat and simmer, covered, for
   30 minutes or until the cauliflower is fairly soft.
3. Stir in the green beans and cook for another 5 minutes or
   so until tender. Season with salt to taste and scatter with the
   coriander leaves before serving.

Wild Rice and Puy Lentils with Lemon and Asparagus

Wild rice is only distantly related to ordinary rice, and it's particularly
rich in protein and minerals. The protein is enhanced by Puy lentils,
which have a good savoury flavour. This dish is great served with a
red onion, tomato, avocado and basil salad. It's good for entertaining,
so the recipe serves 6, but if there are any leftovers they can be
stored in the fridge and eaten the next day. The rice and lentils are
soaked for 4 hours to reduce the cooking time.

Serves 6
GL per serving: 12

250g wild rice
150g dried Puy lentils
1 tsp vegetable bouillon powder
2 courgettes, very thinly sliced lengthways
8 spring onions, trimmed
200g fine asparagus spears
juice of 4 lemons and grated zest of 2 lemons
4 tbsp light olive oil
4 tbsp extra virgin olive oil
salt and freshly ground black pepper

1. Put the rice and lentils in a large saucepan and pour boiling water over them. Cover and leave to soak for 4 hours. Drain in a colander and return the rice and lentils to the saucepan. Add the bouillon powder and pour over 600ml boiling water. Bring to the boil then reduce the heat and simmer for 20 minutes or until cooked and the water has been absorbed.
2. Place the courgette slices in a large bowl with the spring onions and asparagus, and pour the juice of 2 lemons and the light olive oil over them, stirring to coat, then leave to marinate for at least 10 minutes.
3. Preheat a griddle pan until smoking, then griddle the courgette strips very quickly, in batches, turning over to colour on both sides. Add each cooked batch to the pan of cooked rice and lentils. Then griddle the spring onions for 4–5 minutes, rolling them occasionally to colour evenly, then add to the rice and lentils. Next, griddle the asparagus. Put them on the griddle pan – you will probably have to do this in batches – and cook for 5 minutes, rolling them occasionally to cook evenly. Pour a few tablespoons of the leftover marinade into the griddle pan to par-steam the asparagus for a further 1–2 minutes until soft. Add the asparagus to the rice and lentils.

4. Fold the griddled vegetables into the rice and lentils, along with the zest and juice of the remaining 2 lemons and the extra virgin olive oil. Season to taste with salt and pepper. Serve warm or at room temperature.

Baked Bhajis

This healthier, baked version of the Indian classic uses fibre- and protein-rich chickpeas, rather than stodgy potato, plus spinach. These bhajis are delicious as a light lunch or you can serve them with a curry, such as the Lentil and Squash Curry (page 222) or the Chickpea and Cauliflower Curry (page 223), and a little brown basmati rice. Serve with a large wedge of lemon per person to squeeze over the bhajis to bring out the flavour.

Serves 4
GL per serving: 7

2 tbsp ground flaxseed
1 tbsp light olive oil
2 red onions, diced
2 garlic cloves, crushed
4 tsp curry powder
150g baby leaf spinach
2 × 400g cans chickpeas, rinsed and drained
2 heaped tbsp finely chopped fresh coriander leaves
1 tsp salt

1. Put the flaxseed in a small bowl and add 90ml of cold water. Leave to soak for 20 minutes. Preheat the oven to 180°C/350°F/ Gas 4 and line a baking tray with baking paper.
2. Heat the oil in a small saucepan over a medium heat, add the onions and garlic and cook with the curry powder for 5 minutes

or until the onion is softened. Add the spinach to the pan and stir to wilt for a further 1 minute or so.

3. Put the onion mixture in a food processor or blender and add the chickpeas, coriander leaves and salt. Whiz until fairly smooth and combined. Mix in the soaked flaxseed, then shape into 16 patties and put on the prepared baking tray.

4. Cook the bhajis in the oven for 25 minutes or until firm to the touch. Serve.

Tip
Suitable for freezing.

Spiced Cashew and Carrot Burgers

These burgers are absolutely delicious and are packed with fibre and protein. They can be served in wholemeal pitta breads and/or with salad.

Serves 2
GL per serving: 11

1 tbsp ground flaxseed
100g red lentils, rinsed and drained
1 sweet potato, unpeeled, diced
1 tbsp coconut oil or light olive oil
1 garlic clove, crushed
1 red onion, chopped
1 celery stick, finely sliced
1 carrot, finely sliced
50g cashew nuts
1 tsp ground cumin
1 tsp ground coriander
1 tsp sea salt
freshly ground black pepper

1. Put the flaxseed in a small bowl and add 3 tablespoons of cold water. Leave to soak for 20 minutes. Put the lentils and sweet potato in a saucepan over a medium heat and just cover with water. Bring to the boil, then reduce the heat and simmer, covered, for 15 minutes or until just soft (do not allow them to get mushy – you want them to hold their shape as much as possible).

2. Meanwhile, preheat the oven to 200°C/400°F/Gas 6 and line a baking tray with baking paper. Heat the oil in a small frying pan over a medium heat, add the garlic, onion, celery and carrot, and cook for 5 minutes or until softened.

3. Put the onion mixture in a food processor and add the lentils and sweet potato, the cashew nuts, cumin, coriander and salt. Blend until fairly smooth and combined. Season with pepper, mix in the flaxseed and shape into 4 patties. Put on the baking tray and cook for 40 minutes or until slightly coloured on top and firm to the touch.

Tip
Suitable for freezing.

Puy Lentils with Porcini Mushrooms and Thyme

This unusual dish combines interesting flavours and textures from the Puy lentils, which retain their bite after cooking, and the meaty, smoky porcini mushrooms with the aromatic scent of thyme. The lentils and walnuts provide protein, and the fibre content of this dish is also very high.

Serves 2
GL per serving: 6

25g dried porcini mushrooms
200g dried Puy lentils or 400g can cooked lentils, rinsed and drained

1 tbsp light olive oil
2 garlic cloves, crushed
1 red onion, chopped
1 celery stick, finely chopped
2 leeks, finely chopped
50g walnut pieces, roughly chopped
leaves from 1 tbsp fresh thyme sprigs, or to taste
1 tsp sea salt
freshly ground black pepper

1. Put the porcini in a bowl and add warm water to cover. Leave to soak for 30 minutes. Drain in a sieve, reserving the liquid to cook the lentils. Put the dried lentils in a saucepan and add three times the volume of water and the porcini liquor. Bring to the boil, then reduce the heat and simmer, covered, for 25 minutes or until tender. Drain in a colander.
2. Meanwhile, heat the oil in a frying pan over a medium heat, add the garlic, onion, celery and leeks and cook for 2 minutes, then cover and cook for a further 5 minutes or until softened.
3. Add the cooked dried lentils or the canned lentils to the pan of cooked vegetables, then the soaked mushrooms and the walnuts. Stir to combine. Add the thyme and seasoning. Heat through and serve.

Wild Rice Salad with Rosemary Roasted Vegetables

This dish is delicious and filling served simply with a mixed leaf salad. This recipe makes a lot, but leftovers make a wonderfully easy lunch the next day – store in the fridge. Wild rice takes longer to cook than regular rice, but soaking it beforehand reduces the cooking time enormously.

Serves 6
GL per serving: 8

250g wild rice
150g dried Puy lentils
2 courgettes, cut into bite-sized chunks
2 red onions, cut into wedges
2 red, yellow or orange peppers, deseeded and cut into bite-
    sized chunks
4 whole garlic cloves
2 tbsp oil from the jar of sun-blush tomatoes or light olive oil
2 sprigs of rosemary
1 tsp vegetable bouillon powder
100g pitted Kalamata olives, roughly chopped
20 pieces sun-blush tomato, roughly chopped
a good handful basil leaves, torn or chopped
juice of a lemon
salt and freshly ground black pepper

1. Put the wild rice and lentils in a large saucepan and pour boiling
   water over them. Cover and leave to soak for 4 hours or
   until softened.
2. Preheat the oven to 180°C/350°F/Gas 4. Put the courgettes,
   onions, peppers and garlic in a roasting tin and drizzle with the
   oil from the jar of tomatoes, stir to coat evenly, then put the
   rosemary on top. Roast for 45 minutes–1 hour, taking the tray
   out and stirring halfway through to turn the vegetables.
3. After 30 minutes cooking time for the vegetables, drain the
   soaked rice and lentils in a colander, then return them to the
   saucepan with the bouillon powder. Add 600ml boiling water.
   Bring to the boil, then reduce the heat and simmer, covered, for
   20 minutes or until cooked and the water has been absorbed.
4. When the vegetables are cooked (they should be soft when
   pierced), remove the stalks from the rosemary and discard.
   Fold the vegetables into the cooked rice and lentils and stir in
   the remaining ingredients. Season with salt and pepper to taste
   and serve.

Quinoa Salad with Olives, Tomatoes and Pine Nuts

This delicious dish is very quick and easy to make and provides plenty of protein, calcium and zinc. Quinoa is a good source of complete protein for vegans and is quick to cook. A mixed green salad goes well with this.

Serves 4
GL per serving: 9

300g quinoa, rinsed
1 tsp salt
75g pitted Kalamata olives, roughly chopped
100g pine nuts or roughly chopped walnut halves
125g sun-blush tomatoes in olive oil, roughly chopped
2 tbsp oil from the jar of sun-blush tomatoes or light olive oil
100g young spinach leaves, finely chopped
a handful of basil leaves, finely chopped
juice of ½ lemon, or to taste
freshly ground black pepper

1. Put the quinoa in a large saucepan, cover with double the amount of water and add the salt, then bring to the boil. Reduce the heat and simmer, covered, for 12–15 minutes until the water is absorbed and the grains are soft and fluffy.
2. Stir in the olives, pine nuts, tomatoes and the oil, spinach, basil and lemon juice. Season to taste with black pepper and serve.

Chickpea and Spinach Curry

This is an incredibly quick and easy recipe for when time or energy are in short supply. It contains plenty of fibre to make it filling. You could omit the fresh chilli for a milder flavour.

Serves 2
GL per serving: 8

1 tbsp coconut oil or light olive oil
1 red onion, sliced
½ mild red chilli, deseeded and finely chopped
1 tbsp mild or medium curry powder or Madras spice blend
75ml vegetable stock
250ml full-fat coconut milk
400g can chickpeas, rinsed and drained
1 tsp sea salt, or to taste
100g baby leaf spinach, chopped

1. Heat the oil in a large saucepan over a medium heat, add the onion and cook for 3–4 minutes until softened. Add the chilli and curry powder and cook for a further 1 minute.
2. Stir in the stock, coconut milk and chickpeas. Bring to the boil, then reduce the heat and simmer for 15 minutes to reduce the sauce and allow the flavours to combine. Season with salt and taste to check the flavour.
3. Two minutes before you want to serve, stir in the spinach and let it warm through.

Side dishes

Baked Fennel

Slow-roasting fennel brings out its wonderful sweetness and softens the aniseed flavour. This goes well with tomato-based dishes.

Serves 2
GL per serving: 3

2 fennel bulbs, sliced lengthways into quarters
4 tsp lemon juice
2 tbsp light olive oil
salt and freshly ground black pepper

Preheat the oven to 200°C/400°F/Gas 6. Put the fennel in a roasting tin and sprinkle with the lemon juice, oil and seasoning. Cover the tin with foil and bake for 45 minutes or until soft. Serve.

Cannellini Bean Mash

Serve this beany mash with a sauce-based meal. It adds protein and is also satisfying to eat – like mashed potato but healthier.

Serves 2
GL per serving: 5

400g can cannellini beans, rinsed and drained
1 tbsp soya milk or nut milk
1 tsp vegetable bouillon powder
1 tbsp extra virgin olive oil
freshly ground black pepper

1. Put the beans in a blender or food processor and whiz to roughly purée.
2. Transfer to a saucepan over a medium heat and add the remaining ingredients. Heat through, mashing it until fairly smooth. Serve.

Avocado Potato Salad

Mashed avocado makes a great substitute for mayonnaise in this creamy salad – plus it contains far healthier fats.

Serves 2
GL per serving: 5

100g baby new potatoes, scrubbed clean
½ tsp vegetable bouillon powder
½ ripe avocado
1 tbsp lemon juice
½ tbsp finely chopped fresh flat-leaf parsley leaves
freshly ground black pepper

1. Boil the potatoes in a saucepan of water with the bouillon powder for 10–15 minutes until tender. Drain in a colander and then return the potatoes to the pan.
2. Put the avocado in a small bowl and add the lemon juice. Mash with a fork. Add to the pan with the potatoes and stir well. Sprinkle with the parsley and black pepper, and serve.

Spicy Cherry Tomato Potato Salad

This fiery, Spanish-inspired potato salad is best served warm.

Serves 2
GL per serving: 6

100g baby new potatoes, scrubbed clean
¼ tsp vegetable bouillon powder
½ tbsp coconut oil or light olive oil
1 garlic clove, crushed
¼ mild red chilli, deseeded and finely chopped
½ tsp paprika
2 tbsp tomato passata
½ handful cherry tomatoes, halved
½ tsp xylitol
½ tbsp finely chopped fresh flat-leaf parsley leaves

2 spring onions, sliced on the diagonal
freshly ground black pepper

1. Boil the potatoes in in a saucepan of water with the bouillon powder for 10–15 minutes until tender. Drain in a colander and then return the potatoes to the pan.
2. While the potatoes are cooking, heat the oil in a saucepan over a medium heat, add the garlic, chilli and paprika and gently cook for 2 minutes.
3. Add the passata, the cherry tomatoes and the xylitol. Simmer, covered, for 10 minutes.
4. Pour the tomato sauce into the pan with the potatoes. Season with black pepper and sprinkle over the parsley and spring onions. Stir together and serve warm.

Roasted Butternut Squash with Shallots

This great partnering of butternut squash and shallots cooks down to a wonderful melt-in-the-mouth squidginess. Like all orange fruit and vegetables, the squash is a good source of beta-carotene, which your body converts into vitamin A.

Serves 2
GL per serving: 8

½ small butternut squash, peeled, deseeded and cut into bite-sized chunks
8 shallots
1 tbsp light olive oil
freshly ground black pepper

1. Preheat the oven to 200°C/400°F/Gas 6. Put the squash and shallots in a roasting tin and drizzle with oil, shaking them around to coat evenly.

2. Roast for 1 hour, shaking the tray halfway through. The squash is ready when it is fairly soft when pierced with a knife. Remove from the oven, season with black pepper and serve.

Sweet Potato and Carrot Mash

This beautiful orangey mash is rich in flavour and beta-carotene. It is far more sophisticated than mashed potato, but it is just as satisfying. Leaving the sweet potatoes unpeeled preserves more of the nutrients and fibre, but you could peel them if you prefer.

Serves 2
GL per serving: 10

1 sweet potato, unpeeled and sliced thinly
1 carrot, sliced thinly
½ tsp vegetable bouillon powder
freshly ground black pepper

1. Put the sweet potato and carrot in a steamer basket over boiling water and steam for 12 minutes or until soft. Drain the pan and tip the sweet potato into the pan.
2. Mash roughly, then stir in the bouillon powder and pepper, and warm through gently. Serve.

Flageolet Beans in White Sauce

The delicate flavour of flageolet beans is often unfairly overlooked in favour of more robust varieties such as kidney beans. In France they are rightly very popular, however. Here, they are delicious served in a creamy white sauce and are a good protein booster as well as an accompanying vegetable.

Serves 2
GL per serving: 9

2 portions of Tahini White Sauce (see page 204)
400g can flageolet beans, rinsed and drained

Make the sauce according to step 3 of the recipe instructions on page 204. Stir the beans into the sauce in a pan and heat through gently. Serve.

Celeriac and Potato Rösti

Using celeriac to replace some of the potato in this rösti recipe reduces the starch to give it a lower GL. Leaving the skins on the potatoes also serves to lower the impact on blood sugar levels by adding fibre. This is a good dish to accompany a protein dish using nuts, for example.

Serves 2
GL per serving: 7

½ celeriac, peeled
4 small, waxy potatoes, such as Maris Pier, unpeeled
leaves from 3 fresh thyme sprigs
1 tbsp virgin rapeseed oil
salt and freshly ground black pepper

1. Either grate or use a mandolin to produce fine matchsticks of the celeriac and potatoes. Put in a colander over a bowl.
2. Add salt and pepper to the mixture and leave for 5–10 minutes to allow the moisture to drain.
3. Transfer the mixture to a clean tea towel or a piece of muslin. Wrap and twist the fabric to wring out as much liquid as possible. Put the mixture in the fridge for 5 minutes, then repeat the process. Stir in the thyme.

4. Heat the oil in a frying pan over a medium heat and add the mixture, either as one large cake or use rings to make smaller cakes. Aim for a thickness of 1–2.5cm. Fry until brown, then reduce the heat to low and cook for 8 minutes each side, or until the mixture is cooked through.

Braised Kale with Almonds

Braising kale in bouillon makes it wonderfully soft and well flavoured, with the almonds providing a little crunch. Kale is, of course, a cruciferous vegetable and its dark green colour shows how rich it is in phytonutrients.

Serves 2
GL per serving: 1

50g flaked almonds
1 tbsp coconut oil
1 garlic clove, crushed
1 tsp vegetable bouillon powder
115g curly kale, stems removed, leaves sliced
freshly ground black pepper

1. Toast the almonds in a dry frying pan over a low heat for a few minutes or until lightly browned, taking care not to let them burn.
2. Add the oil and swirl it around the pan to coat (take the pan off the heat temporarily to stop it from burning), then throw in the garlic, and stir.
3. Put the bouillon in a small bowl and add 4 tablespoons of hot water. Stir to dissolve. Add the kale and bouillon to the pan, stir, then cover and allow to steam-fry for 2 minutes or until the kale is tender. If the pan runs dry, add a little more water. Season with black pepper, then serve.

Steam-frying

You can cook a variety of vegetables in this way, giving them lots of flavour. The great advantage of steam-frying is that the lower temperature of steaming doesn't destroy nutrients in the way that frying does, and you use only a very small amount of oil, if that. Use a shallow saucepan or a deep frying pan with a thick base and a lid that seals well. You can steam-fry without oil by first adding 2 tablespoons of liquid to the pan – this can be water, vegetable stock, soy sauce or a little watered-down sauce that you'll use for the dish. Once it boils, immediately add some vegetables, then cook rapidly for 1–2 minutes, turn up the heat, add 1–2 tablespoons more of the liquid and clamp the lid on tightly. After 1 minute, add the remaining ingredients. Turn the heat down after 2 minutes and steam in this way until the vegetables are al dente.

Alternatively, add 1 teaspoon to 1 tablespoon olive oil or coconut oil to the pan, warm it, add the ingredients and cook. After 2 minutes, add 2 tablespoons of liquid as above and clamp the lid on. Steam the ingredients until the vegetables are al dente.

Indian Spiced Butternut Squash

The bright orange flesh of squashes shows that they are high in the antioxidant beta-carotene. Squash provides plenty of fibre, vitamins and slow-releasing, low-GL energy. Serve this as a side dish with curries to complete the protein element.

Serves 4
GL per serving: 7

800g butternut squash, unpeeled
½ tsp ground turmeric
1½ tsp ground cumin
1½ tsp ground coriander
2 tbsp tomato purée
1 tbsp light olive oil
salt and freshly ground black pepper

1. Preheat the oven to 200°C/400°F/Gas 6. Cut the butternut squash in half lengthways and scrape out the seeds and pulp with a spoon. Cut again into eighths, so that you have eight long pieces in total.
2. Put the turmeric in a bowl and add the cumin, coriander, tomato purée and oil. Mix together, then rub the paste all over the squash until evenly coated. Season with salt and pepper.
3. Put the squash in a roasting tin and cook for 45–60 minutes until the flesh is soft when pierced or squashed, turning the pieces over halfway through cooking. Serve.

Peperonata

This is absolutely delicious – soft, sweet, slow-roasted peppers, onions and tomatoes with a flavour kick from the olives. Peperonata is the perfect addition to a cold lunch of hummus and green salad.

Serves 4
GL per serving: 5

75ml light olive oil
6 garlic cloves, sliced

2 red onions, thinly sliced into wedges
2 red peppers, deseeded and thinly sliced lengthways
2 yellow or orange peppers, deseeded and thinly sliced lengthways
225g cherry tomatoes
100g Kalamata olives, pitted if you prefer
1 tsp sea salt
freshly ground black pepper
1 tbsp fresh basil leaves, roughly torn

1. Heat the oil in a large saucepan over a medium heat, add the garlic and onions and cook for 10 minutes or until softened.
2. Add the peppers, cover and cook for a further 10 minutes, then add the tomatoes and olives. Cook for a further 15–20 minutes until the tomatoes soften and burst, and all the vegetables are soft. Season with the salt and pepper and scatter with the basil. Serve warm or at room temperature.

Soy and Sesame Steam-fried Tenderstem Broccoli

Broccoli contains protein as well as folate and choline and makes a good accompaniment to any dish.

Serves 4
GL per serving: 0.5

1 tsp vegetable bouillon powder
1 tsp cornflour
1 tbsp toasted sesame oil
1 tbsp tamari or soy sauce
200g Tenderstem broccoli
1 tbsp coconut oil or light olive oil

1. Put the bouillon in a cup and add the cornflour, sesame oil, soy sauce and 2 tablespoons of water. Mix well.

2. Cut the broccoli spears into thirds. Heat the coconut oil in a wok or a large saucepan over a medium heat. Add the broccoli and stir-fry for 2 minutes, then soak a sheet of kitchen paper in cold water and put this over the broccoli, to cover the pan. Put the lid on and steam-fry for 2 minutes or until the vegetables soften a little.

3. Pour in the sauce and allow it to come to the boil, to coat the broccoli and cook the cornflour. Serve.

Herbed Puy Lentils

The quantities and ingredients for this recipe are very adaptable – simply throw in whichever fresh herbs and leaves you have to hand to create a refreshing, vitamin C-packed salsa verde-style mixture. This side dish salad also contains protein to add to a lighter main course, and you can stir in some toasted pine nuts or pumpkin seeds for extra flavour, if you like.

Serves 4
GL per serving: 4

300g dried Puy lentils
75g watercress
150g baby leaf spinach
25g fresh basil leaves
25g fresh flat-leaf parsley leaves
1 large garlic clove, crushed
juice of 2 lemons, or to taste
4 tbsp extra virgin olive oil, or to taste
salt and freshly ground black pepper

1. Put the lentils in a large saucepan and add 1 teaspoon of sea salt. Cover with boiling water, bring to the boil, then reduce the heat and simmer, covered, for 20 minutes or until the lentils are

cooked. Drain in a colander and set aside to cool while you make the herby sauce.

2. Put the leaves in a food processor or blender and add the herbs, garlic, lemon juice, oil and black pepper. Whiz to chop finely.
3. Stir the leaf mixture into the cooked and cooled lentils and taste to check the flavour – add more lemon, oil or pepper or add some salt, if you like.

Tip
This mixture is also perfect stirred through wild rice or brown rice.

Vinaigrette

Using two types of oil and some herbs makes this dressing a little tastier than the standard vinaigrette.

Makes about 250ml
GL per serving: 1

100ml extra virgin olive oil
100ml virgin pumpkin seed oil, avocado oil or rapeseed oil
2 tbsp cider vinegar
4 tsp balsamic vinegar
1 garlic clove, crushed
1 tsp Dijon mustard
½ tsp xylitol
1 tsp herbes de Provence
salt and freshly ground black pepper

Put all the ingredients in a screw-topped jar and shake it to emulsify them. Taste and adjust the seasoning.

Tahini Dressing

This nutty dressing has the creamy texture of mayonnaise, but has a punchier taste and contains beneficial fats from the tahini, sesame and olive oil, as well as plenty of antioxidant nutrients. Use to dress salad leaves for added flavour and nutrients.

Serves 2
GL per serving: 1

1 tbsp tahini
1 garlic clove, crushed
2 tbsp extra virgin olive oil
1 tsp sesame oil
1 tsp finely chopped fresh flat-leaf parsley leaves
½ tsp ground cumin
2 tsp lemon juice
freshly ground black pepper

Put all the ingredients in a small bowl and mix well together until smooth. Serve.

Lemon and Garlic Dressing

This simple dressing, with the classic Mediterranean flavours of lemon and garlic, makes green salads much more interesting.

Serves 2
GL per serving: 1

4 tbsp extra virgin olive oil
1 tbsp lemon juice
1 tsp Dijon mustard
1 garlic clove, crushed

a pinch of xylitol
a good pinch of paprika
a good pinch of curry powder
a good pinch of dried herbes de Provence
salt and freshly ground black pepper

Put all the ingredients in a small bowl or screw-top jar and mix well together. Adjust the seasoning to taste and serve.

Oriental Dressing

This will give flavour to steam-fries (see page 239), stir-fries and fresh soba noodles. Fresh ginger is extremely good for you as it has strong anti-viral and anti-inflammatory properties. It also contains zinc, which is essential for immune function, so it is a good idea to include it in your diet as much as possible.

Serves 2
GL per serving: 1

2 tsp sesame oil
2 tbsp tamari or soy sauce
2cm root ginger, peeled and grated
2 garlic cloves, crushed
2 tsp mirin (Japanese rice cooking wine)

Put all the ingredients in a small bowl or screw-top jar and add 4 tablespoons of cold water. Mix together, then serve.

Sweet treats

Cacao and Almond Cake

Delicious, moist and filling, this is a great treat for afternoon tea. Alternatively, you could serve it as a dessert with vegan ice cream (there are now some wonderful coconut- and nut-based ones available) or simply with berries. It's packed with minerals and antioxidants.

Makes 10 slices
GL per serving: 9 per slice (half that if you use agave syrup)

3 tbsp ground flaxseed
coconut oil, for greasing
200g ground almonds
50g cacao powder or cocoa powder
150ml light olive oil or virgin rapeseed oil
125ml maple syrup or agave syrup
1 tsp ground cinnamon
2 tsp vanilla extract
½ tsp bicarbonate of soda

1. Put the flaxseed in a bowl and add 125ml cold water. Leave to soak for 20 minutes to thicken.
2. Preheat the oven to 190°C/375°F/Gas 5 and grease a 20cm cake tin. Put the remaining ingredients in a large mixing bowl and combine. Add the soaked flaxseed and stir until smooth.
3. Spoon the mixture into the prepared tin and bake for 30 minutes or until fairly firm on top. Leave to cool for 5 minutes in the tin and then transfer to a wire rack to cool completely. Store in an airtight container.

Tip
Suitable for freezing.

Lemon and Blueberry Cake

Using olive oil instead of butter, and a binding agent of soaked flaxseed, this cake is a vegan version of a classic favourite, combining lemon and blueberries. The GL is a little high but you can have a smaller slice if it'll take you over your GL target for the day. This recipe can be made with a good quality gluten-free flour as well as standard self-raising.

Makes 10 slices
GL per serving: 15 per slice

2 tbsp ground flaxseed
375g self-raising flour
125ml light olive oil or virgin rapeseed oil
125ml oat milk or other plant-based milk
juice and grated zest of 3 lemons
150g fresh blueberries
2 tbsp xylitol

1. Put the flaxseed in a small bowl and add 90ml water. Leave to soak for 20 minutes to thicken.
2. Preheat the oven to 190°C/375°F/Gas 5 and line a 20cm cake tin with baking paper.
3. Put the remaining ingredients in a mixing bowl and mix well, then stir in the soaked flaxseed to bind the mixture together.
4. Spoon into the prepared tin and bake for 40–45 minutes or until the cake is golden, firm and springy to the touch and not too wobbly. Leave to cool in the tin for 5 minutes and then turn out onto a wire rack to cool. Enjoy it warm or leave to cool completely. Store in an airtight container and eat within 2 days.

Tip

Suitable for freezing.

Because the top is crisp and the centre moist, it's easier to cut the cake into appropriate-sized slices using a bread knife.

Chocolate, Beetroot and Hazelnut Slices

Beetroot is often used in chocolate cake recipes because it gives the crumb a lovely moist texture. You don't notice the beetroot at all, but it adds fibre and goodness. This recipe can be made with a good quality gluten-free flour as well as standard self-raising.

Makes 16 slices
GL per serving: 3

2 tbsp ground flaxseed
125g vacuum-packed cooked beetroot (not in vinegar) or
   2 beetroot, cooked and peeled
100g hazelnuts, coarsely chopped
50g cacao powder or cocoa powder
200ml agave syrup (or maple syrup but it will increase the GL)
125ml oat milk
125ml light olive oil or virgin rapeseed oil
325g self-raising flour
1 tsp ground cinnamon (optional)
1 tsp vanilla extract

1. Put the flaxseed in a small bowl and add 90ml cold water. Leave to soak for 20 minutes to thicken.
2. Preheat the oven to 180°C/350°F/Gas 4 and line a 22cm square cake tin with baking paper.
3. Put all the ingredients in a food processor and whiz until well combined and smooth. (Alternatively, to mix by hand, grate the beetroot and then mix with all the other ingredients.)

4. Spoon the mixture into the cake tin and bake for 15–20 minutes or until firm to the touch. Cut into 16 slices while still in the tin, then leave on a wire rack to cool completely before removing from the tin.

Almond Custard

Enhance stewed or baked fruit with this dairy-free alternative to traditional custard. It's just as smooth and delicious, and the use of almonds means it contains some protein too.

Serves 2
GL per serving: 2

1 level tbsp cornflour
1 heaped tbsp ground almonds
1 heaped tbsp xylitol

1. Put the cornflour in a bowl and add 2 tablespoons of water. Mix until smooth.
2. Pour this mixture into a small saucepan and add the ground almonds and xylitol. Heat gently, stirring constantly, for 5 minutes, while gradually adding 180ml water to form a smooth, thick sauce. Serve.

Almond Shortbread

Rich and wonderfully crumbly, shortbread is a much-loved biscuit – but it usually gets its richness from butter. This vegan version uses protein-rich quinoa flour to raise the protein level and makes ample use of ground nuts. The result is even crumblier than the traditional version, and just as mouthwatering.

Serves 2 (2 each)
GL per serving: 4

25g coconut oil, at room temperature
25g xylitol
25g ground almonds
50g quinoa flour
1 handful of flaked almonds

1. Preheat the oven to 170°C/325°F/Gas 3 and line a small baking tray with baking paper. If the coconut oil is still hard, heat it very slightly to soften it. Put the coconut oil and xylitol in a mixing bowl and beat using an electric whisk until light and creamy.
2. Rub the ground almonds and quinoa flour into the mixture using your fingertips, working lightly – the mixture should soon resemble breadcrumbs.
3. Press the mixture evenly into the prepared baking tin to form a square about 1cm thick (don't worry that it doesn't cover the entire tray), sprinkle with flaked almonds and bake for 20 minutes.
4. Allow to cool on a wire rack, then cut into 4 squares.

Tip
Store in an airtight container for up to 3 days.

Chocolate Crunchies

This is a brilliant standby for when you have unexpected guests. Make a batch, cut it up and keep it in the freezer. It can be served from frozen, which makes it wonderfully chewy and a little like a chocolate ice cream bar. It might taste decadent, but the ingredients are all very nutritious – the dark chocolate included.

Serves 10
GL per serving: 8

200g dairy-free dark chocolate (70 per cent cocoa solids), broken into chunks

125g rough oatcakes
50g goji berries
50g Brazil nuts, roughly chopped
50g pumpkin seeds
4 tsp ground mixed spice
2 tsp ground cinnamon
50g hazelnut butter or unsalted peanut butter

1. Line a baking sheet with baking paper. Melt the chocolate, stirring occasionally, in a heatproof bowl over a pan of gently simmering water, making sure the base of the bowl doesn't touch the water.
2. Put the oatcakes into a mixing bowl and crumble into small pieces. Stir in the goji berries, nuts, seeds and spices.
3. Stir the hazelnut butter into the melted chocolate and mix until smooth. Stir the chocolate mixture into the dry ingredients, making sure the ingredients are evenly coated.
4. Spread the mixture over the prepared baking sheet and put in the fridge or freezer to chill and harden. Break into 10 shards or cut into rough pieces when set, ready to serve.

Tip
Suitable for freezing.

Coconut and Pineapple Sorbet

Sweet, creamy and delicious with fresh fruit such as berries or mango, this is a Caribbean-inspired ice cream-meets-sorbet affair. Pineapple is the perfect food to end a meal with as it contains bromelain, an enzyme that digests protein, to help you break down your food.

Serves 6–8
GL per serving: 3

275g fresh pineapple, or canned pineapple in juice, drained
1 tbsp xylitol
juice of a lime
400ml can full-fat coconut milk
100g desiccated coconut

1. Put the pineapple into a blender or food processor and add the xylitol and lime juice. Whiz together until you have a purée. Stir or blend in the coconut milk, then stir in the desiccated coconut.
2. Pour into a freezer-proof container and freeze for 1 hour, until it's just setting at the edges, then beat well or blend again. Return it to the freezer for at least another 4 hours or overnight, until it's set solid.
3. Remove from the freezer 20–30 minutes before serving to allow it to soften a little, then blend in a food processor to create a thick, creamy consistency and remove any remaining ice crystals (the lack of cream means that it's harder when frozen than dairy ice cream). Alternatively, use an ice cream maker and follow the manufacturer's instructions. You can also serve this sorbet while it's still slushy.

Coconut Oat Biscuits

The ground ginger in this recipe gives the biscuits a warming flavour. Agave syrup comes from the cactus plant and is a useful vegan alternative to honey. It has a naturally low GL, which means that it won't send your blood sugar levels soaring, but it is high in fructose so it's important to go easy on it.

Makes 10
GL per serving: 6

75g coconut oil or dairy-free margarine suitable for baking
25g xylitol

1 tbsp agave syrup
100g whole rolled oats
50g desiccated coconut
1–2 tsp ground ginger, to taste

1. Preheat the oven to 170°C/325°F/Gas 3. Line a baking tray with baking paper. Put the oil and xylitol in a small saucepan over a medium-low heat and add the syrup. Melt and dissolve together, taking care not to let it boil. Stir in the oats, coconut and ginger.
2. Shape the mixture into ten walnut-sized balls. The mixture will be very crumbly at this stage, so press it together firmly before putting the biscuits on the prepared baking tray.
3. Bake for 20 minutes or until they're just turning golden on top. Leave on a wire rack to harden and cool.

Tip
Suitable for freezing.

Banana Flapjack Bites

These soft, chewy biscuits are naturally free from wheat, refined sugar and added fat. They get all their sweetness from the banana and agave syrup and their soft texture from the banana and the tahini paste.

Makes 6
GL per serving: 4

2 tbsp agave syrup
2 tbsp tahini
100g whole rolled oats
50g ground almonds
1 ripe banana, mashed

1. Preheat the oven to 170°C/325°F/Gas 3. Line a baking tray with baking paper. Mix all the ingredients together in a mixing bowl to form a sticky mixture.
2. Shape into six balls and put on the prepared baking tray. Bake for 25–30 minutes until just turning golden on top. Leave on a wire rack to harden and cool.

Tip
Suitable for freezing.

Applejack Slices

These soft, moist slices of apple flapjack are rich in soluble fibre and make a delicious teatime treat.

Serves 8
GL per serving: 4

2 Bramley apples
150g coconut oil
4 tbsp agave syrup
200g whole rolled oats
100g ground almonds
100g xylitol
4 tsp ground mixed spice or ground cinnamon (optional)

1. Preheat the oven to 170°C/325°F /Gas 3. Line a 20cm cake tin with baking paper. Core the apples, but don't peel them, then coarsely grate them. Gently stew the grated apple in a little water in a saucepan for 2 minutes or until softened. Add the oil plus the syrup and melt together, taking care not to let the mixture boil. Stir in the oats, almonds, xylitol and spice.
2. Spoon the mixture evenly into the cake tin, then bake for 30 minutes or until just turning golden on top. Leave on a wire

rack to harden and cool before slicing and storing in an airtight container.

Apricot and Ginger Flapjack Bites

Apricots are a good source of fibre and they are also rich in beta-carotene. Choose unsulfured ones, which are not bright orange, if you wish to avoid preservatives.

Makes 10
GL per serving: 4

50g dried unsulfured apricots
75g stem ginger in syrup, drained
75g coconut oil
1 tbsp agave syrup
100g whole rolled oats
50g ground almonds

1. Preheat the oven to 170°C/325°F/Gas 3. Line a baking tray with baking paper. Very finely chop the apricots and ginger to make a mushy paste (or whiz in a food processor or blender). Put it in a small saucepan over a medium-low heat. Add the oil and syrup, and gently melt, taking care not to let it boil.
2. Stir in the oats and almonds to coat evenly. Allow to cook slightly.
3. Shape the mixture into 10 walnut-sized balls and put on the prepared baking tray. Bake for 20 minutes or until just turning golden on top. Leave on a wire rack to harden and cool.

Tip
Suitable for freezing.

Plum Crumble with Cinnamon and Oats

This sticky, sweet, proper pud uses oats and almonds for a healthier crumble topping, rather than flour.

Serves 6
GL per serving: 8

200g jumbo oats
100g ground almonds
50g xylitol
100g coconut oil

Filling:
1kg plums, halved and stoned
3 tsp ground cinnamon
50g xylitol

1. Preheat the oven to 180°C/350°F/Gas 4. Put half the oats in a food processor and whiz to grind into flour. Add the ground almonds, xylitol and coconut oil and blitz again to form crumbs. Stir in the remaining oats.
2. For the filling, put the plums in the base of a baking dish. Scatter with the cinnamon and xylitol, top with the crumble mixture and even out the surface. Bake for 40–50 minutes until the top starts to turn golden brown and the fruit is soft. Serve warm.

Tip
Suitable for freezing.

Chapter 11

Supplements for Optimum Health

M ost people don't realise why supplementation, for everyone, not just vegans, is needed to achieve what our bodies and brains had access to throughout our evolution from primate to man. Our ancestors expended much more energy than we do so they had to eat more in order to sustain themselves. What they ate had to be fresh, organic and whole. There were no fridges, refining and processing. Analyses of what we used to obtain in the way of nutrients, even as recently as the Victorian age, show that the only way we could achieve the same level of nutrients today would be to either supplement or fortify foods.

In previous chapters you learnt that plant-based foods alone do not provide sufficient vitamin B12, vitamin D (in the winter) and omega-3 EPA and, especially, DHA as well as choline. In addition, while a plant-based, wholefood, organic diet is sufficient and rich in many nutrients, some minerals can also be tricky. Among these are the minerals that are plentiful in seafood, and in food grown in or near the sea, such as selenium and iodine. Iodine and selenium, for example, are found richly in kelp and other sea-weeds. While vegetables and fruit tend to be rich in magnesium and potassium, seeds and nuts are rich in calcium and zinc, and beans and other pulses are rich in iron, these mineral concentrations depend much more on what's in the soil than the inherent properties of the plant. Organic farming aims, as a principle, to re-mineralise the soil, but, even so, it is not so easy to know what level of nutrients you're getting.

Another nutrient that is not easily obtained from diet in quantities sufficient for optimal health is vitamin C. This is because we, like all primates, lost the ability to make vitamin C during, one supposes, a period of evolution where we lived in a vitamin C-rich, jungle-type environment. Primates who still live in such an environment eat *a lot* of vitamin-C: gorillas, for example, consume between 2,000 and 4,000mg a day, while most monkeys eat over 500mg a day, which is six times the basic RNI (Reference Nutrient Intake) of 80mg. For we humans, taking in over 500mg, and possibly 2 grams a day, equates to optimal health in terms of the lowest risk of related diseases such as infections and cardiovascular disease. The average person achieves an intake of around 100mg, which means that many are below this level. An orange provides approximately 50mg so, to achieve an intake of say 1 gram a day, we'd need to eat 20 oranges! But all that sugar, without the amount of exercise our ancestors used to take, would make us fat.

Recognising the challenges in meeting optimal nutrient intake, a wise vegan would take four supplements:

- A high-strength 'optimum' multivitamin and mineral that provides, together with other nutrients, 10mcg of B12, 15mcg of vitamin D, and iodine, selenium and iron.
- Extra vitamin C – 1 to 2 grams.

- Essential omega-3 fats providing EPA (200–300mg) and DHA (200–300mg), or combined EPA+DHA to 500mg. The most critical target is to achieve 250mg of DHA.
- Choline, from lecithin granules (1 tbsp) or capsules (2–3 capsules) or a supplement providing 200–500mg.

All of these nutrients are available from vegan sources.

Since many of these nutrients, especially the water-soluble vitamins B and C, are excreted by the body within six hours you make better use of them by dividing the dose, for example, taking a multivitamin and mineral twice a day, rather than all these amounts once a day. This is what I do, taking four supplements twice a day.

In Resources on pages 262–3 I give examples of supplements that fulfil these requirements.

Taking these, together with eating in line with the guidelines in Parts 1 and 2, and the recipes in Part 3, is your best strategy for vegan superhealth!

Resources

Foods

Clearspring sell a wide range of sea vegetable products, including SeaVeg Crispies (dried nori), which are a natural source of selenium and iodine. Their products are widely available in health food stores and online at www.clearspring.co.uk

Pulsin sell a natural pea protein powder (as well as vanilla and chocolate flavoured varieties) that is low GL and great for vegan shakes. They also have soya and rice protein powders. Their Plant-based Keto Bar is the lowest GL bar I've found and comes in a range of flavours (my favourite is the chocolate fudge and peanut flavour). They are widely available in health food shops or online at www.pulsin.co.uk.

Nibble Protein make high-protein, low-GL snacks. The Lemon Nibble Protein Bites have the lowest GL. There are six bites per 42g bag and each bite is about 1g of sugar, or 6g per bag, plus 10g of protein. They are available from www.nibbleprotein.com

Blueberry Active and **Cherry Active** are highly concentrated juices. Mix a 30ml serving with 250ml water to make a deliciously healthy, low-GL cherry or blueberry juice. Each 946ml bottle of Cherry Active contains the juice from over 3,000 cherries – that's half a tree's worth – and contains a month's supply. Blueberry Active is made with 100% premium quality blueberries. Each serving is packed full of blueberries and contains no added sugars, sweeteners, preservatives, colourings or flavourings. Available online at www.HOLFORDirect.com and https://active-edge.co.uk/

Engevita Nutritional Yeast Flakes with Added B12 is available from good health food stores and Amazon.

Supplements

Patrick Holford has formulated a range of supplements to support optimal health, which are available from HOLFORDirect. com. All his supplements are certified vegan, except for Essential Omegas, which contain fish oil, and fish gelatin capsules.

Multivitamin and mineral supplements

The backbone of a supplement programme is a high-strength optimum multivitamin and mineral, with extra vitamin C and essential fats, especially omega-3 DHA.

Essentials4Vegans is a combination of the four nutrients that are hardest to get on a vegan diet, namely vitamin B12, vitamin D, omega-3 DHA and the phospholipid choline. Taking two vege-caps a day provides these four nutrients in optimal amounts:
Vitamin B12 10mcg
Vitamin D3, derived from lichen, 400iu (10mcg)
Omega-3 DHA 250mg
Choline 200mg

Taken twice a day together with Patrick Holford's certified-vegan Optimum Nutrition Formula, which is a comprehensive multi-vitamin and mineral providing calcium (300mg), magnesium (155mg), iron and zinc (each 10mg), selenium and iodine (each 30mcg); and vitamin D (15mcg or 600iu) and ImmuneC, comprehensively covers all nutrients required for optimal health, supported by a wholefood diet.

Other good multivitamins include Solgar's Vegetarian Multiple (with vitamin D3 400iu) and Viridian's Vegan Multi (with vitamin D3 400iu). You will also need to supplement extra DHA, choline and D3, especially in the winter. Most multis provide 400iu but you want to aim for 1,000iu of vitamin D in the winter and to support healthy immunity. See solgar.co.uk and viridian-nutrition.com for details of suppliers and online purchase.

The Vegan Society sells a supplement, VEG1, that provides basic levels of B12 (25mcg), B2 (1.2mg), B6 (2.2mg), D3 (20mcg or 800iu), folic acid (200mcg), iodine (150mcg) and selenium (60mcg) but no omega-3 or phospholipids. Available from www.vegansociety.com.

Get Up & Go with Carboslow® is a combination of vitamins, minerals, essential fats, protein and fibre, and is designed to be mixed into a tasty vegan shake. One serving is just 8 GLs and is perfect for those following a low-GL, slow-carb diet. There is no need to take a multivitamin and mineral if you have Get Up & Go since it provides optimal levels of most vitamins and minerals. However, it does not provide sufficient omega-3 DHA, choline and vitamin D so it is still worth supplementing Essentials4Vegans or a similar product.

Nutritional information

The Pernicious Anaemia Society If you feel very tired on a vegan diet and/or suspect you might be lacking vitamin B12 The Pernicious Anaemia Society is a useful resource. The charity's website has a lot of useful information and a list of symptoms. Those with pernicious anaemia need more B12 than others due to an inability to effectively absorb B12 from food and convert it into the active form. I use their symptom check in my 100% Health Check (see below). If you fill in this questionnaire and come up lacking in B12, find out more at their website https://pernicious-anaemia-society.org.

100% Health Check You can have your own personal health and nutrition assessment online using Patrick Holford's 100% Health Check. This gives you a personalised assessment of your current health, and what you most need to change. Visit www.patrick-holford.com and go to 'FREE health check'. If, after completing the 100% Health Check, you join the 100% Health Club you'll get a 40-page report, and unlimited access to help you address your needs as your health improves. You also receive Patrick Holford's 100% Health newsletter every other month, plus instant access to all past newsletters online; special reports each month (and access to his library of hundreds of reports on important health issues); a hotline to use via the private 100% Health members Facebook group; 20 per cent off most seminars and events; up to 30 per cent off all books and supplements from HOLFORDirect.com (up to 15 per cent on foods); and a free copy of a Patrick Holford book on joining. Membership costs £7.99 a month.

The Vegan Society provides a wealth of information about topics pertinent to being vegan, including nutritional issues and local events. Go to www.vegansociety.com.

The Food for the Brain Foundation is a non-profit educational charity, founded by Patrick Holford, which aims to promote awareness of the link between learning, behaviour, mental health and nutrition; and to educate and provide educational material to children, parents, teachers, schools, the public, the catering industry, health professionals and the government. The website has a free Cognitive Function Test. It takes 15 minutes to complete. If you are at all concerned about your cognition this test is well worth taking. Depending on your score, it tells you what to do to improve your memory. For more information visit www.foodforthebrain.org.

Nutritional therapy

BANT, the British Association of Nutrition and Lifestyle Medicine, is the official register of qualified nutritional therapists. You can search for a therapist by area and see their specialisms should you need support with any health issues. See www.bant. org.uk. In Ireland see the Nutritional Therapists of Ireland at www.ntoi.ie

The Institute for Optimum Nutrition (ION), founded by Patrick Holford, offers a three-year diploma course in nutritional therapy. Visit www.ion.ac.uk, address: Ambassador House, Paradise Road, Richmond TW9 1SQ, UK, tel.: +44 (0)20 8614 7815

Tests

Food intolerances YorkTest Laboratories have a self-test kit for identifying food intolerances, called Food Scan. The FoodScan 113 identifies the foods causing the intolerance and the level of intolerance. In addition, the service includes nutritionist consultations and comprehensive support and advice on managing your elimination diet. To order call YorkTest Laboratories on 0800 130

0580 or visit www.yorktest.com. Use the code PH10 to get a 10% discount on the website or by calling their number.

Homocysteine can be tested using a home test kit from www.yorktest.com or call 0800 130 0580. Use the code PH10 to get 10% discount on the website or by calling their number.

Liver function can be tested using a home test kit measuring two liver enzymes called AST and ALT. This is available from www.yorktest.com as part of their Essential Health Check. Use the code PH10 to get 10% discount on the website or by calling their number.

Vitamin D testing is usually available through your doctor. Alternatively, you can be tested for £29, using a home test kit for blood collection, which is then sent back to the laboratory. See www.vitamindtest.org.uk. It is also part of Yorktest's Essential Health Check, along with foliate, B12 and iron. Use the code PH10 to get a 10% discount.

Patrick's retreats and events

Want to totally transform your health? Spend three days with Patrick for a new you, transforming mind, body and spirit. Patrick's three-day **Total Health Transformation** is an immersive experience in a magical setting of Fforest Barn Mountain retreat, only 2.5 hours from London or Manchester. You'll learn how to transform your health with Patrick's seven health secrets, simple exercises to balance your body and mind, become a kitchen wizard, reconnect with your true self, and feel energised and vibrant. The retreats happen twice a year, in May and September, in small groups. We cater for vegans. See www.patrickholford.com/events for details.

Go keto, detox and rejuvenate with Patrick Holford, following his **5-Day Diet**, then two days low GL at his Fforest Barn Mountain retreat in South Wales. These 7-day 'Hybrid Fast Detox' retreats happen twice a year, in May and September. We cater for vegans. For details on the next retreats visit www.patrickholford. com/events.

The above retreat is followed by a three-day **Vegan, Plant-based Cookery Retreat**, at Fforest Barn, with chefs Mike and Sam Thomsett teaching participants how to prepare and enjoy delicious plant-based meals based on Patrick Holford's optimum nutrition principles. See www.patrickholford.com/events for details.

Patrick regularly speaks at events in the UK and Ireland. For details of his upcoming events go to www.patrickholford.com/ events.

Facebook and Instagram

Stay involved with the conversation about health and nutrition on my Facebook page https://www.facebook.com/patrickholford/; Instagram – patrickholford.uk

Further reading

The Hybrid Diet, Patrick Holford and Jerome Burne, Piatkus (2018)
The Optimum Nutrition Bible, Patrick Holford, Piatkus (1998)
The Ten Secrets of 100% Healthy People, Patrick Holford, Piatkus (2009)
The Low-GL Diet Bible, Patrick Holford, Piatkus (2009)

Notes

1. The Principles of Optimum Nutrition

1   Benton, D. and Roberts, G., 'Effect of vitamin and mineral supplementation on intelligence sample of schoolchildren', *Lancet* (Jan 1988); 1(8578): 140–3.

2   Taitt, H. et al., 'Global trends and prostate cancer: a review of incidence, detection, and mortality as influenced by race, ethnicity, and geographic location', *American Journal of Men's Health* (Nov 2018); 12(6): 1807–1823. doi: 10.1177/1557988318798279

3   Ghoncheh, M. et al., 'The incidence and mortality and epidemiology of breast cancer in the world', *Asian Pacific Journal of Cancer Prevention*, vol. 17, Cancer Control in Western Asia Special Issue, 201643 doi: 10.7314/APJCP.2016.17.S3.43.

4   Rizzi, L. et al., 'Global epidemiology of dementia: Alzheimer's and vascular types', *Biomed Research International* (2014); 908915. doi: 10.1155/2014/908915.

5   See www.diabetes.org.uk/about_us/news/new-stats-people-living-with-diabetes.

6   See www.diabetes.org/resources/statistics/statistics-about-diabetes.

7   See www.gov.uk/government/news/flu-vaccine-effectiveness-in-2017-to-2018-season; *see also*, for 2019 statistics, Kissling, E. et al., 'Interim 2018/19 influenza vaccine effectiveness: six European studies, October 2018 to January 2019', *Eurosurveillance* (Feb 2019); 24(8): 1900121. doi: 10.2807/1560-7917.

8   Castillo-Fernandez, J.E. et al., 'Epigenetics of discordant monozygotic twins: implications for disease', *Genome Medicine* (Jul 2014); 6(7): 60. doi: 10.1186/s13073-014-0060-z.

9   Read *Say No to Cancer* by Patrick Holford for a fuller discussion of this topic.

10 Ko, K. et al., 'Dietary intake and breast cancer among carriers and noncarriers of BRCA mutations in the Korean Hereditary Breast Cancer Study', *American Journal of Clinical Nutrition* (Dec 2013); 98(6): 1493–501. doi: 10.3945/ajcn.112.057760; *see also* Romagnolo, D. et al., 'Genistein prevents BRCA1 CpG methylation and proliferation in human breast cancer cells with activated aromatic hydrocarbon receptor', *Current Developments in Nutrition* (May 2017); 1(6): e000562. doi: 10.3945/cdn.117.000562.

11 Bekris, L. et al., 'Genetics of Alzheimer disease', *Journal of Geriatric Psychiatry and Neurology* (Dec 2010); 23(4): 213–27. doi: 10.1177/0891988710383571.

12 Hemilä, H. 'Vitamin C and infections', *Nutrients* (Mar 2017); 29;9(4). pii: E339. doi: 10.3390/nu9040339. Review.

13 Clayton, P. et al., 'An unsuitable and degraded diet?: public health lessons from the mid-Victorian working class diet', *Journal of Royal Society of Medicine* (2008): 101: 282–89. Doi: 10.1258/jrsm.2008.080112 285.

14 See www.bbc.co.uk/news/health-39057146.

2. Choosing a More Plant-Based Diet Makes Good Health Sense

1 https://www.pnas.org/content/pnas/early/2018/03/20/1713820115.full. pdf. Shepon, A. et al., 'The opportunity cost of animal-based diets exceeds all food losses', *PNAS* (Apr 2018); 115(15): 3804–9. doi/10.1073/pnas.1713820115.

2 Oyebode, O., Gordon-Dseagu, V. and Walker A, et al., 'Fruit and vegetable consumption and all-cause, cancer and CVD mortality: analysis of health survey for England data', *Journal of Epidemiology and Community Health* (2014); 68: 856–62.

3 Fraser, G. 'Vegetarian diets and cardiovascular risk factors in black members of the Adventist health study', *Public Health Nutrition* (2015); 18(3): 537–45.

4 Lee, Y. and Park, K., 'Adherence to a vegetarian diet and diabetes risk: a review and meta-analysis of observational studies', *Nutrients* (Jun 2017); 9(6): 603.; *see also* Chiu, T. 'Vegetarian diet, change in dietary patterns, and diabetes risk: a prospective Study', *Nutrition & Diabetes* (2018); 8: 12.

5 Malik, V. et al., 'Dietary protein intake and risk of type 2 diabetes in US men and women', *American Journal of Epidemiology* (Apr 2016); 183(8): 715–28.

6 Barnard, N. et al., 'A low-fat vegan diet and a conventional diabetes diet in the treatment of type 2 diabetes: a randomized, controlled, 74-wk clinical trial', *American Journal of Clinical Nutrition* (May 2009); 89(5): 1588S–1596S. doi: 10.3945/ajcn.2009.26736H.

7 Fraser, G. et al., 'Lower rates of cancer and all-cause mortality in an Adventist cohort compared with a US census population', *Cancer* (Mar 2020); 126(5): 1102–11. doi: 10.1002/cncr.32571.

8 Dinu, M. et al., 'Vegetarian, vegan diets and multiple health outcomes: a systematic review with meta-analysis of observational studies', *Critical Reviews in Food Science and Nutrition* (Nov 2017); 57(17): 3640–9. doi: 10.1080/10408398.2016.1138447.

9 Penniecook-Sawyers, J. et al., 'Vegetarian dietary patterns and the risk of breast cancer in a low-risk population', *British Journal of Nutrition* (May 2016); 115(10): 1790–7. doi: 10.1017/S0007114516000751.

10 Najjar, R. et al., 'Defined, plant-based diet utilized in an outpatient cardiovascular clinic effectively treats hypercholesterolemia and hypertension and reduces medications', *Clinical Cardiology* (Mar 2018); 41(3): 307–13.

11 Rohrmann, S. et al., 'Meat consumption and mortality –results from the European prospective investigation into cancer and nutrition', *BMC Medicine* (2013); 11: 63. doi: 10.1186/1741-7015-11-63.

12 Micha, R. et al., 'Association between dietary factors and mortality from heart disease, stroke, and type 2 diabetes in the United States', *JAMA* (Mar 2017); 317(9): 912–24.

13 Schwingshackl, L. et al. 'Comparison of high vs. normal/low protein diets on renal function in subjects without chronic kidney disease: a systematic review and meta-analysis', *PLoS One* (May 2014); 9(5): e97656.

14 Della Guardia, L. et al., 'Insulin sensitivity and glucose homeostasis can be influenced by metabolic acid load', *Nutrients* (May 2018); 10(5).

15 Donaldson, M., 'Nutrition and cancer: a review of the evidence for an anti-cancer diet', *Nutrition Journal* (Oct 2004); 3: 19.

16 See https://www.wcrf.org/sites/default/files/Meat-Fish-and-Dairy-products.pdf

17 Schwingshackl, L. et al., 'Food groups and risk of colorectal cancer', *International Journal of Cancer* (May 2018); 142(9): 1748–58.

18 Brinkworth, G. et al., 'Long-term effects of a very low-carbohydrate diet and a low-fat diet on mood and cognitive function', *Archives of Internal Medicine* (2009); 169(20): 1873–80.

19 Ganmaa, D. et al., 'Incidence and mortality of testicular and prostatic cancers in relation to world dietary practices', *International Journal of Cancer* (Mar 2002); 98(2): 262–7.

20 Ibid.

21 Ibid.

22 Chan, J.M. et al., 'Plasma insulin-like growth factor-I and prostate cancer risk: a prospective study', *Science* (1998); 279(5350): 563–66.

23 Stanford, J.L. et al., *Prostate cancer trends 1973–1995*, Bethesda, MD: National Cancer Institute (1999).

24   Chan, J.M. et al., 'Dairy products, calcium, and prostate cancer risk in
     the physicians' health study', *American Journal of Clinical Nutrition*
     (2001), 74(4): 549–54. *See also* Stanford, J.L. et al., *Prostate cancer trends
     1973–1995*, Bethesda, MD: National Cancer Institute (1999); Krogh, P.V.
     'Meat, eggs, dairy products, and risk of breast cancer in the European
     prospective investigation into cancer and nutrition (EPIC) cohort',
     American Journal of Clinical Nutrition (2009); 90(3): 602–12; LeRoith, D.
     and Roberts Jr., C.T., 'The insulin-like growth factor system and cancer',
     Cancer Letters (2003); 195(2):127–137; Hankinson, S.E. et al., 'Circulating
     concentrations of insulin-like growth factor-I and risk of breast cancer',
     Lancet (1998); 351(9113): 1393–6; Wu, M.H. et al., 'Relationships between
     critical period of estrogen exposure and circulating levels of insulin-like
     growth factor-I (IGF-I) in breast cancer: evidence from a case-control
     study', *International Journal of Cancer* (2010); 126(2): 508–14; Chan, J.M.
     et al., 'Plasma insulin-like growth factor-I and prostate cancer risk: a
     prospective study', *Science* (1998); 279(5350): 563–6; Giovannucci, E. et al.,
     'Calcium and fructose intake in relation to risk of prostate cancer', *Cancer
     Research* (1998); 58(3): 442–7.

25   Synnove, K. et al., 'Dairy, soy, and risk of breast cancer: those confounded
     milks', *International Journal of Epidemiology* (Feb 2020); 25: ii: dyaa007.
     doi: 10.1093/ije/dyaa007.

26   van der Pols, J.C. et al., 'Childhood dairy intake and adult cancer risk:
     65-y follow-up of the Boyd Orr cohort', *American Journal of Clinical
     Nutrition* (2007); 86(6): 1722–9.

27   Vogel, K. et al., 'The effect of dairy intake on bone mass and body
     composition in early pubertal girls and boys: a randomized controlled
     trial', *American Journal of Clinical Nutrition* (May 2017); 105(5): 1214–29.
     doi: 10.3945/ajcn.116.140418.

28   Tai, V. et al., 'Calcium intake and bone mineral density: systematic review
     and meta-analysis', *British Medical Journal* (Sep 2015); 351:h4183. doi:
     10.1136/bmj.h4183. Review.

29   Holford, P. and Trustram-Eve, C., '100 per cent Health's Digestion
     Survey', Holford & Associates 2017 – free download from www.
     patrickholford.com/digestion.

30   Reddy, S. et al., 'Faecal pH, bile acid and sterol concentrations in
     premenopausal Indian and white vegetarian compared with white
     omnivores', *British Journal of Nutrition* (1998); 79: 495–500.

31   Hambly, R. et al., 'Effects of high- and low-risk diets on gut microflora-
     associated biomarkers of colon cancer in human flora associated rats',
     Nutrition and Cancer (1997); 27(3): 250–5.

3. Nutrients are Team Players

1   Schoenthaler, S. et al., 'Controlled trial of vitamin-mineral supplementation on intelligence and brain function', *Personality and Individual Differences* (1991);12(4): 343–50; Schoenthaler, S. et al., 'Controlled trial of vitamin-mineral supplementation: effects on intelligence and performance', *Personality and Individual Differences* (1991), 12(4): 351–62.

2   Gesch, B., 'The SCASO Project', *International Journal of Biosocial Medical Research* (1990); 12(1): 41–68.

3   Koyama, K. et al., 'Efficacy of methylcobalamin on lowering total homocysteine plasma concentrations in haemodialysis patients receiving high-dose folate supplementation', *Nephrology, Dialysis, Transplantation: Official Publication of the European Dialysis and Transplant Association* (2002); 17: 916–22.

4. Anti-Nutrients – the Dark Side of Nutrition

1   Cave, M. et al., 'Polychlorinated biphenyls, lead, and mercury are associated with liver disease in American adults: NHANES 2003-2004' *Environmental Health Perspectives* (Dec 2010); 118(12): 1735–42; Younossi, Z.M. et al., 'Changes in the prevalence of the most common causes of chronic liver diseases in the United States from 1988 to 2008', *Clinical Gastroenterology and Hepatology* (Jun 2011); 9(6): 524–530.e1; Lee, H. et al., 'Associations between blood mercury levels and subclinical changes in liver enzymes among South Korean general adults: analysis of 2008–2012, Korean national health and nutrition examination survey data', *Environmental Research* (Apr 2014); 130: 14–9; Min, Y.S., Lim, H.S. and Kim H., 'Biomarkers for polycyclic aromatic hydrocarbons and serum liver enzymes', *American Journal of Industrial Medicine* (Jul 2015); 58(7): 764–72; Lin, C.Y. et al., 'Investigation of the associations between low-dose serum perfluorinated chemicals and liver enzymes in US adults', *American Journal of Gastroenterology* (Jun 2010); 105(6): 1354–63.

2   Guallar E, et al., 'Confounding of the relation between homocysteine and peripheral arterial disease by lead, cadmium, and renal function', *American Journal of Epidemiology* (Apr 2006); 163(8): 700–08.

3   Schectman, G. et al., 'Ascorbic acid requirements for smokers: analysis of a population survey', *American Journal of Clinical Nutrition* (1991); 53(6): 1466–70.

4   Pirmohamed, M. et al., 'Adverse drug reactions as cause of admission to hospital: prospective analysis of 18,820 patients', *British Medical Journal* (Jul 2004); 329(7,456): 15–9.

5. How to Get Enough Protein

1 Schwingshackl, L. and Hoffmann, G. 'Comparison of high vs. normal/low protein diets on renal function in subjects without chronic kidney disease: a systematic review and meta-analysis', *PLoS One* (2014); 9(5): e97656.

2 My book *Say No Cancer* (2010) gives the evidence for the association of milk and soya and hormone-related cancers.

3 Messina, M. and Redman, G. 'Effects of soy protein and soybean isoflavones on thyroid function in healthy adults and hypothyroid patients: a review of the relevant literature', *Thyroid* (Mar 2006); 16(3): 249–58.

4 Fraser, G. 'Vegetarian diets and cardiovascular risk factors in black members of the Adventist health study,' *Public Health Nutrition* (2015); 18(3): 537–45.

5 Lee, Y. and Park, K., 'Adherence to a vegetarian diet and diabetes risk: a review and meta-analysis of observational studies', *Nutrients* (Jun 2017); 9(6): 603.; *see also* T. Chiu 'Vegetarian diet, change in dietary patterns, and diabetes risk: a prospective Study', *Nutrition & Diabetes* (2018); 8: 12.

6 Malik, V. et al., 'Dietary protein intake and risk of type 2 diabetes in US men and women', *American Journal of Epidemiology* (Apr 2016); 183(8): 715–28.

6. The Importance of 'Brain' Fats

1 Ogundipe E, et al., 'Randomized controlled trial of brain specific fatty acid supplementation in pregnant women increases brain volumes on MRI scans of their newborn infants', *Prostaglandins, Leukotrienes and Essential Fatty Acids* (Nov 2018);138: 6–13. doi: 10.1016/j.plefa.2018.09.001.

2 Craddock J, et al., 'Algal supplementation of vegetarian eating patterns improves plasma and serum docosahexaenoic acid concentrations and omega-3 indices: a systematic literature review', *Journal of Human Nutrition and Dietetics*. (Dec 2017); 30(6): 693–9. doi: 10.1111/jhn.12474.

3 Elorinne A, et al., 'Food and nutrient intake and nutritional status of Finnish vegans and non-vegetarians', *PLoS One* (2016); 11(2): e0148235. doi: 10.1371/journal.pone.0148235

4 Burdge, G. et al., 'Metabolism of alpha-linolenic acid in humans', *Prostaglandins, Leukotrienes and Essential Fatty Acids* (Sep 2006); 75(3): 161–8.

5 Emken, E, et al., *Biochimica Biophysica Acta* (1994);1213: 277–288.

6 Ailsa Welch study: https://academic.oup.com/ajcn/article/92/5/1040/4597496

7 Zatonski, W. et al., 'Rapid declines in coronary heart disease mortality in

Eastern Europe are associated with increased consumption of oils rich in alpha-linolenic acid', *European Journal of Epidemiology* (2008); 23(1): 3–10.

8   Campos, H. et al., 'Alpha-linolenic acid and risk of nonfatal acute myocardial infarction', *Circulation* (Jul 2008); 118(4): 339–45. doi:10.1161/CIRCULATIONAHA.107.762419.

9   Pinto, A. et al., 'A comparison of heart rate variability, n-3 PUFA status and lipid mediator profile in age- and BMI-matched middle-aged vegans and omnivores', *British Journal of Nutrition* (Mar 2017); 117(5): 669–85. doi: 10.1017/S0007114517000629.

10 Ogundipe, E. et al., 'Peri-conception maternal lipid profiles predict pregnancy outcomes', *Prostaglandins, Leukotrienes and Essential Fatty Acids* (Nov 2016); 114: 35–43. doi: 10.1016/j.plefa.2016.08.012.

11 Olsen, S. et al., 'Plasma concentrations of long chain n-3 fatty acids in early and mid-pregnancy and risk of early preterm birth', *EBioMedicine* (2018); 35: 325–33.

12 Kofod Vinding, R. et al., 'Fish oil supplementation in pregnancy increases gestational age, size for gestational age, and birth weight in infants: a randomized controlled trial', *Journal of Nutrition* (2019); 149(4): 628–34. https://doi.org/10.1093/jn/nxy204.

13 Bernard, J.Y. et al., 'Maternal plasma phosphatidylcholine polyunsaturated fatty acids during pregnancy and offspring growth and adiposity', *Prostaglandins, Leukotrienes and Essential Fatty Acids* (Jun 2017); 121: 21–29. doi: 10.1016/j.plefa.2017.05.006.

14 Ogundipe, E. et al., 'Randomized controlled trial of brain specific fatty acid supplementation in pregnant women increases brain volumes on MRI scans of their newborn infants', *Prostaglandins, Leukotrienes and Essential Fatty Acids* (Nov 2018); 138: 6–13. doi: 10.1016/j.plefa.2018.09.001.

15 Hibbeln, J. et al., 'Maternal seafood consumption in pregnancy and neurodevelopmental outcomes in childhood (ALSPAC study): an observational cohort study', *Lancet* (Feb 2007); 369(9561): 578–85.

16 Gould, J et al., 'Seven-year follow-up of children born to women in a randomized trial of prenatal DHA supplementation', *JAMA* (2017); 317(11): 1173–75. doi:10.1001/jama.2016.21303. 35, 651–667

17 dos Santos Vaz, J. et al., 'Dietary patterns, n-3 fatty acids intake from seafood and high levels of anxiety symptoms during pregnancy: findings from the Avon longitudinal study of parents and children', *PLoS One* (2013); 8(7): e67671.

18 Derbyshire, E., 'Could we be overlooking a potential choline crisis in the United Kingdom?', *BMJ Nutrition, Prevention and Health*, (2019); 0:1–4.

19 Pyapali, G. et al., 'Prenatal dietary choline supplementation decreases the threshold for induction of long-term potentiation in young adult rats', *Journal of Neurophysiology* (Apr 1998);7 9(4): 1790–6.

20 Caudill, M. et al, 'Maternal choline supplementation during the third trimester of pregnancy improves infant information processing speed: a randomized, double-blind, controlled feeding study' *FASEB Journal* (Apr 2018); 32(4): 2172-80. doi: 10.1096/fj.201700692RR.

21 Bahnfleth, C. et al., 'Prenatal choline supplementation improves child color-location memory task performance at 7 years of age (FS05-01-19)', *Current Developments in Nutrition* (2019), 3 (Suppl. 1). doi: 10.1093/cdn/nzz052.FS05-01-19.

7. Control Your Sugar and Energy

22 Bao, J. et al., 'Prediction of postprandial glycemia and insulinemia in lean, young, healthy adults: glycemic load compared with carbohydrate content alone', *American Journal of Clinical Nutrition* (May 2011); 93(5): 984–96; *see also* Krog-Mikkelsen, I. et al., 'A low glycemic index diet does not affect postprandial energy metabolism but decreases postprandial insulinemia and increases fullness ratings in healthy women', *Journal of Nutrition* (Sep 2011); 141(9): 1679–84.

23 Cheraskin, E., 'The breakfast/lunch/dinner ritual', *Journal of Orthomolecular Medicine* (1993); 8(1): 6–10.

24 Paoli, A. et al., 'The influence of meal frequency and timing on health in humans: the role of fasting', *Nutrients* (Mar 2019) 28; 11(4).

25 Braaten, J. et al, 'High beta-glucan oat bran and oat gum reduce postprandial blood glucose and insulin in subjects with and without type 2 diabetes', *Diabetic Medicine* (1994); 11(3): 312–18.

8. Vitamin Essentials

1 Yajnik C, et al., 'Vitamin B12 deficiency and hyperhomocysteinemia in rural and urban Indians', *Journal of the Association of Physicians of India* (2006); 54: 775–82.

2 Pawlak, R., et al., 'Vitamin B-12 content in breast milk of vegan, vegetarian, and nonvegetarian lactating women in the United States', *American Journal of Clinical Nutrition* (Sep 2018); 108(3): 525–31.

3 Damayanti, D. et al., 'Foods and supplements associated with vitamin B12 biomarkers among vegetarian and non-vegetarian participants of the Adventist health study-2 (AHS-2) calibration study', *Nutrients* (Jun 2018);10(6).

4 Vogiatzoglou, A. et al, 'Vitamin B12 status and rate of brain volume loss in community-dwelling elderly', *Neurology* (2008); 71: 826–32.

5 Watanabe, F. et al., 'Vitamin B12-containing plantfood sources for vegetarians', *Nutrients* (2014); 6:1861–73.

6   Watanabe, F. and Bito, B., 'Vitamin B12 sources and microbial interaction', *Experimental Biology and Medicine* (2018); 243: 148–158. doi: 10.1177/1535370217746612.

7   Yamada, K. et al., 'Bioavailability of dried asakusanori (*porphyra tenera*) as a source of cobalamin (vitamin B12)', *International Journal for Vitamin and Nutrition Research* (1999); 69: 412-18. https://doi. org/10.1024/0300-9831.69.6.412.

8   Bito, T. et al., 'Characterization and quantitation of vitamin B12 compounds in various chlorella supplements', *Journal of Agricultural and food Chemistry* (Nov 2016); 64(45): 8516–24.

9   Merchant, R. et al., 'Nutritional supplementation with chlorella pyrenoidosa lowers serum methylmalonic acid in vegans and vegetarians with a suspected vitamin B12 deficiency', *Journal of Medicinal Food* (Dec 2015); 18(12): 1357–62. doi: 10.1089/jmf.2015.0056.

10   Watanabe, F. et al., 'Pseudovitamin B(12) is the predominant cobamide of an algal health food, spirulina tablets', *Journal of Agricultural and Food Chemistry* (Nov 1999); 47(11): 4736–41.

11   Madhubalaji, C. et al., 'Improvement of vitamin B12 status with spirulina supplementation in Wistar rats validated through functional and circulatory markers', *Journal of Food Biochemistry* (Nov 2019); 43(11): e13038.

12   Dagnelie, P. et al., 'Vitamin B-12 from algae appears not to be bioavailable', *American Journal of Clinical Nutrition* (1991); 53: 695–7.

13   See https://www.b12-vitamin.com/algae/

14   Miyamoto, E. et al., 'Purification and characterization of a corrinoid-compound in an edible cyanobacterium Aphanizomenon flos-aquae as a nutritional supplementary food', *Journal of Agricultural and Food Chemistry*, (2006), 54. Jg., Nr. 25, S. 9604–7.

15   Teng, F. et al., 'Vitamin B12[c-lac-tone], a biologically inactive corrinoid compound, occurs in cultured and dried lion's mane mushroom (*Hericium erinaceus*) fruiting bodies', *Journal of Agricultural and Food Chemistry* (2014); 62: 1726–32.

16   Schwarz, J. et al., 'The influence of a whole food vegan diet with nori algae and wild mushrooms on selected blood parameters', *Clinical Laboratory* (2014); 60(12): 2039–50. https://www.ncbi.nlm.nih.gov/pubmed/25651739.

17   Nakos, M. et al., 'Isolation and analysis of vitamin B12 from plant samples', *Food Chemistry* (Feb 2017); 216: 301–8. doi: 10.1016/j. foodchem.2016.08.037.

18   Bischoff-Ferrari, H., 'Optimal serum 25-hydroxyvitamin D levels for multiple health outcomes', *Advances in Experimental Medicine and Biology* (2014); 810: 500–25. doi:10.1007/978-1-4939-0437-2_28; *see also* Pludowski, P, et al., 'Vitamin D supplementation guidelines', *Journal of*

Steroid Biochemistry and Molecular Biology (Jan 2018); 175: 125–35. doi: 10.1016/j.jsbmb.2017.01.021.

19   Cardwell, G. et al., 'A Review of mushrooms as a potential source of dietary vitamin D', *Nutrients* (Oct 2018); 10(10): 1498. doi: 10.3390/ nu10101498.

9. The Importance of Minerals

1   Foster, M. et al., 'Effects of vegetarian diets on zinc status: a systematic review and meta-analysis of studies in humans', *Journal of the Science of Food and Agriculture* (Aug 2013); 93(10): 2362–71. doi: 10.1002/jsfa.6179.

2   Foster, M. et al., 'Zinc status of vegetarians during pregnancy: a systematic review of observational studies and meta-analysis of zinc intake', *Nutrients* (Jun 2015); 7(6): 4512–25. doi: 10.3390/nu7064512. https://www.ncbi.nlm.nih.gov/pubmed/26056918.

3   Guillin, O. et al., 'Selenium, selenoproteins and viral infection', *Nutrients* (2019), 11(9): 2101. https://www.mdpi.com/2072-6643/11/9/2101; *see also* Zhang, J. et al., 'Association between regional selenium status and reported outcome of COVID-19 cases in China', *American Journal of Clinical Nutrition* (2020); 00: 1–3. doi/10.1093/ajcn/nqaa095/5826147.

4   Velasco, I. et al., 'Iodine as essential nutrient during the first 1000 days of life', *Nutrients* (2018); 10(3): 290. https://doi.org/10.3390/nu10030290.

Index

Note: page numbers in **bold** refer to diagrams, page numbers in *italics* refer to information contained in tables.

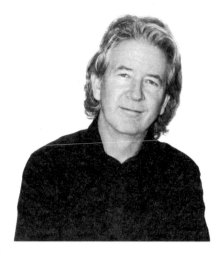

NOT GOOD?

AVERAGE?

REASONABLY HEALTHY?

HEALTHY?

Take my FREE health check right now!

I invite you to take my free online Health Check. You'll get instant results and a practical action plan to transform your health.

This detailed, online questionnaire reviews your diet, lifestyle, and any symptoms you may currently have. It should only take a few minutes to complete. Rest assured participation is entirely free and completely confidential.

The Health Check will give you a current health score between 0-100% and then show you which key areas of your health you can focus on to move towards 100% health. I anticipate you'll see and feel a difference within 30 days. Get started at:

www.patrickholford.com